THE

HOMŒOPATHIC GUIDE,

IN ALL DISEASES

OF THE

URINARY AND SEXUAL ORGANS,

INCLUDING THE DERANGEMENTS CAUSED BY

Onanism and Sexual Excesses;

WITH A STRICT REGARD TO THE PRESENT DEMANDS OF MEDICAL SCIENCE,

AND ACCOMPANIED BY AN APPENDIX

ON THE USE OF

ELECTRO-MAGNETISM

IN THE TREATMENT OF THESE DISEASES,

BY

WM. GOLLMANN, M. D.

TRANSLATED, WITH ADDITIONS,

BY

CHAS. J. HEMPEL, M. D.

Fellow and Corresponding Member of the Homœopathic Medical College of Pennsylvania;
Honorary Member of the Hahnemann Society of London, &c. &c.

PHILADELPHIA:
PUBLISHED BY RADEMACHER & SHEEK, No. 239 ARCH STREET.
NEW YORK:—WILLIAM RADDE, 322 BROADWAY.
1855.

King & Baird, Printers, Sansom Street.

EDITOR'S PREFACE.

Gollmann's work commends itself to the profession, as one of sterling merit in more than one sense. In the first place, it does not deal in unmeaning, incoherent symptoms, but is, throughout, adapted to the present demands of medical science as respects diagnosis, pathology, and a description of all the characteristic pathognomonic signs of disease. And, in the second place, the work is complete; it omits no important or interesting fact, and presents such a classification of the diseases of which it treats, as the rational mind can at once accept as philosophical and satisfactory.

Such a work as Gollmann's will be particularly serviceable to the few superficial and one-sided symptomatists still lagging behind the great body of homœopathic physicians, who are constantly and earnestly pressing forward towards the goal of scientific truth in the treatment of disease. It will convince the reader, provided conviction can at all be impressed upon his mind, that disease is something more than a mere agglomeration of symptoms, and that morbid conditions of the system may arise, where the highest exercise of the reasoning faculty has to be brought into play, in order to determine the real quality of a group of apparent phenomena. How could we ever succeed in successfully treating the various forms of secondary and tertiary syphilis, including almost every variety of disorganisation of the various tissues, if we did not first take the trouble to trace these disorganisations to their first causes, by means of the reasoning faculty guided by the Ariadnean thread of physiology and pathology? Let any physician undertake to treat a syphilitic ulceration of the throat, syphilitic tubercles, exanthems, bone-pains, or syphilitic caries and necrosis, syphilitic iritis, syphilitic epilepsy, or syphilitic cachexia, according to mere symptoms, and then see where such treatment would lead him. Why, the treatment could not even be commenced. The symptomatic treatment of all such diseases is radically impossible. Scarcely any of the symptoms which characterise these diseases, have been reproduced in our provings upon the healthy. In the numerous cases of mercurial poisoning, recorded in the books, a few disorganisations similar to those above named, have indeed, been observed, but they are far, very far, from being sufficiently numerous to serve as a basis for a strict symptomatic treatment. If the treatment of these affections is not conducted according to reason, but simply according to the law of outward or apparent similarity, which is a mere perception on the plane of sense, it will not only remain nugatory, but the poison will run its triumphant career until the organism falls a victim to its virulence. I am well aware that there are still a few ignorant pretenders in the homœopathic school, who reject the existence of all secondary and tertiary forms of the syphilitic disease; in corroboration of this statement, I may here allude to a writer in the Philadelphia Journal of Homœopathy, a certain Adolphus Lippe, who, with a ridiculous boldness, asserted that there was no such a thing as secondary or tertiary syphilis. Homœopathic physicians are getting to be ashamed of the childish assumptions of such scribblers, and, thanks to the more enlightened teachings emanating from individual physicians, from well-organised homœopathic colleges, and from the liberal portion of the allœopathic brotherhood, the time is fast approaching, when homœopathy will no longer be a separate and distinct system of medical treatment, but the true formula of therapeutics, to which all medical truths will tend as naturally as the rivers converge in their common reservoir, the ocean.

Attention is directed to the appendix, on the use of electro-magnetism in the treatment of sexual diseases. I am enabled to corroborate, from personal experience, all that Gollmann says, in praise of this great agent, and my friend, Doctor D. D. Smith, of this city, who is in the habit of combining electro-magnetism with homœopathic treatment, and, for this purpose, uses electro-magnetic lockets, batteries, &c., of his own contrivance, is constantly obtaining the most brilliant results from the use of electro-magnetism in sexual diseases, of any form or degree of intensity.

In Gollmann's work, the symptomatic indications for the use of particular remedies have been omitted. I have supplied them in the present translation, and trust that they will prove an acceptable and useful addition to the original.

CHARLES J. HEMPEL, M. D.,
54 Bond Street.

New York, Sept., 1854.

AUTHOR'S PREFACE.

In giving this work to the public, the author was neither actuated by the desire of enriching the book-trade, nor by the vain glory of being heard in the vast forum of science. He was simply moved by the deep conviction acquired by years of observation and experience, in the exclusive treatment of diseases of the sexual and urinary organs, that these diseases very frequently destroy all domestic happiness; that they cause deep bodily and mental suffering, and prepare for the sufferer a sad and distressing future.

Experience has likewise convinced him, that a satisfactory knowledge of the origin and spread of these diseases, and of the physiological, anatomical and morphological relations of the organs which are the seat of the sexual and urinary functions, will afford to rational and enlightened laymen the most certain means of putting a stop to the spread of these affections.

The author does not mean to imply, however, that he wrote this work for laymen only; on the contrary, he feels confident, that physicians will likewise derive essential advantages from this work, inasmuch as regard has been had to all the demands of modern science, and all the recent physiological, chemical, and pathologico-anatomical discoveries, have been used as a basis in the composition of this treatise.

The author has, therefore, deemed it his duty, with conscientious care and an independent, critical judgment, to combine his own experience, with the knowledge contained in the best and most recent writings concerning the treatment of this disease; he mentions, with gratitude, the names of *Ricord*, *Sigmund*, *Zeisl*, *Wallace*, *Waller*, *Cazenave*, *Hebra*, and others, who have shed such brilliant light on the nature and treatment of syphilitic diseases, and whose thorough investigations and observations in this respect, have constantly served as a basis for his own studies.

This acknowledgment, of course, only applies to the scientific diagnosis, etiology and prognosis of these diseases, not to the treatment. The treatment recommended by the author, is strictly homœopathic, and, on this account, differs considerably, from that proposed by the above-mentioned authors. In describing the treatment, all those remedies have been recommended, which, according to his notes, had been of essential service to the author in the management of these affections. The intelligent reader will at once perceive, that these remedies have been selected with a certain discrimination, and with a strict regard to the actual forms of the disease; whereas, less efficient remedies, or such as only referred to particular symptoms, have been omitted. The particular indications of these few specific remedies had to be left to the judgment of the attending physician, who has to determine what remedies ought to be used in every special case. It is only in diseases where a layman who is sufficiently versed in homœopathy, might safely prescribe for himself, without the interference of a physician, that the principal symptomatic indications have been given. The manner in which these remedies are to be administered, on such occasions, will be found briefly indicated in the subsequent introduction.

The author has deemed it expedient to commence the work with an account of the anatomical structure, and of the physiological functions of the sexual and urinary organs. Considering the high rank, which chemistry and the microscope occupy in modern medicine, the author deemed a chemical analysis of the healthy urine, and a microscopical account of the spermatozoa which play such an important part in the function of propagation, indispensable.

After furnishing these anatomical and physiological details, which are equally important and interesting to the physician and layman, the author enters upon the description of the various diseases. The arrangament which has been followed by him in this respect, requires a short explanation.

The author deemed it expedient to commence this work with a description of the sexual diseases, because they occur more frequently, and are more varied, than others. These diseases are naturally divided into two classes, one of which is composed of the diseases which are communicated by contact generally by being inoculated during the sexual act by means of a virulent matter; the second class comprises the diseases emanating from mechanical causes, congenital malformations, sexual excesses of all kinds.

In the first division, we have treated all such diseases as owe their immediate origin to an impure coït; our classification of these diseases differs somewhat from the views of other authors. Such diseases as cannot be inoculated by means of a contagium, have been ranged under the head of *simple venereal diseases.* These cases have been described by Sigmund, as syphilitic blennorrhagia. To this class of diseases belong the various cases of gonorrhœa, with their direct and indirect consequences.

The second class of this extensive group of diseases, comprises those forms of disease which are endowed with an inoculable poison. These forms of disease are known under the name of *ulcerous syphilis*, termed primary syphilis, as long as the poison has not infected the general organism. From the moment when the poison loses its local action, and, by infecting the blood, developes constitutional symptoms, an essential difference is perceived between these two forms of disease. The disease now becomes a general or constitutional syphilis, which is again distinguished in secondary and tertiary syphilis, each of which is characterised by striking appearances.

The third class is composed of sexual diseases which cannot be traced to a contagium, but which have a great influence on the happiness of mankind, and either weaken or destroy the sexual power. Onanism and sexual excesses, which are the most frequent causes of these diseases, have been dilated upon with particular care, and we recommend this chapter to the attention of our non-professional readers as a means of guarding against a host of distressing maladies.

The *diseases of the urinary organs* form the last part of the work.

The work has been enriched with an appendix on electro-magnetism, which has recently played such an important part in sexual diseases, and which we ourselves have employed in so many cases with distinguished success. In this appendix we have furnished a brief outline of the efficacy of this agent, and of our method of using it; a method, from which we have derived the most brilliant results in the treatment of sexual diseases.

In publishing this work, we have only thought of the weal

of our fellow-beings, and we shall deem ourselves sufficiently rewarded for our trouble, if our efforts should contribute in some slight degree to a limitation of diseases which so seriously impair the welfare of human society.

August, 1853.

INTRODUCTION.

IN order to facilitate the use of this work, we have deemed it appropriate, for the benefit of laymen, to furnish a few indications concerning the use of the agents which are recommended in this work, including rules for a repetition of the dose, and for the alternate exhibition of two or more drugs.

Taking it for granted, that both laymen and physicians are acquainted with the rules according to which homœopathic medicines have to be selected, and more particularly with the fundamental law, that a remedial agent, in order to be homœopathic to a disease, must be capable of producing in the healthy organism, a train of symptoms, similar to those of the disease, we will at once pass over to the practical rules concerning the exhibition of the drug.

As regards the dose, we never go above the sixth or seventh potency. From the commencement of our practice, we have had every reason to prefer this attenuation to any other. We never adhere to one drug, if it is evident that no cure can be expected from it. If one drug fails us, we resort to a second, and even third. It seems to us a reprehensible practice, to adhere to the exclusive use of one drug, if this drug evidently has no effect on the condition of the patient. In obstinate cases, we do not hesitate to combine surgical means with the homœopathic treatment.

Strict regard has to be had to the mental condition of the patient. In some cases, the choice of an otherwise appropriately indicated remedy, is determined by the moral condition of the patient. If the patient is disposed to lowness of spirits, we recommend *Aurum;* if to religious melancholy, *Veratrum;* if to a weeping mood, *Pulsatilla, Ignatia, Sepia;* if of an irritable disposition, *Bryonia,* and if, very nervous, *Coffea.*

Diet and regimen, are of particular importance under homœopathic treatment. The patients ought to abstain from stimulants, spices, fat, and flatulent food, tea, coffee, wine, and all other spirituous drinks. Indigestible food, or food which oppresses the stomach, such as goose, duck, pork, heavy farinaceous diet, pastry, etc., have likewise to be avoided.

The success of a homœopathic treatment is very much interfered with by every thing that excites and disturbs the mind, such as depression of spirits, books, company, or theatrical representations that excite the senses.

A cure is promoted by cheerful surroundings, in the country, or in some open and pleasant part of the city; by moderate bodily exercise, and abstinence from mental exertions. The repetition of the dose depends entirely upon the nature of the case. Dangerous and intensely-acute diseases, which run a rapid course, require a much more frequent repetition of the dose than chronic diseases that run a slow course.

These few indications will probably suffice; in difficult or doubtful cases, a physician will have to be consulted.

SECTION I.

ANATOMICAL AND PHYSIOLOGICAL DESCRIPTION OF THE URINARY AND SEXUAL ORGANS OF THE MALE AND FEMALE.

THE urinary and sexual organs are so closely related to each other, both as respects their original development and the union of their secretory ducts, that, although performing vastly different functions, they may, nevertheless, be treated anatomically as one set of organs. The same organ which serves as an outlet to the urine secreted by the kidneys, is likewise designed to carry, with a feeling of the highest sexual delight, the fructifying semen of the male into the vagina of the female, through which it is transmitted to the inner organs of generation and gestation, where, after a period of forty weeks, the future man, the lord of creation, is developed in a most marvellous manner out of a drop of the male spermatic fluid.

The Urinary Organs.

They consist of pairs of glandular organs which secrete the urine; of their excretory canals, the *kidneys* and *ureters*, and of a single hollow organ in which the urine collects, and which is termed *bladder*, which discharges its contents through the *urethra*.

I. THE KIDNEYS.

The kidneys are two glandular bodies situated in the lumbar region, and designed to secrete the urine. The right kidney is somewhat lower than the left, to accommodate the right lobe of the liver, which is situated above it. Both kidneys are surrounded by a fatty, loose cellular tissue, which keeps them in place. In shape they resemble a bean, the outer border being convex, the inner concave; the latter is provided with a fissure, where the renal vessels enter the organ, on which account this fissure is termed the *gate of the kidneys* or *hilus renalis*. The structure of the parenchyma of the kidney is very curious. If a longitudinal incision is made into the kidney, a whitish triangular substance is discovered with the naked eye, around which we perceive another substance of a brown-red color.

Former anatomists termed the whitish mass the *medullary*, and the brown-red substance the *cortical* substance of the kidneys. But, thanks to the microscope, we now know that the so-called medullary substance consists of an infinite number of delicate tubes termed the *tubes of Bellini;* and that the cortical substance is simply a net-work of vessels, formed by the tortuous convolutions of microscopic twigs of the renal artery, and designated as the *tubes of Ferrein.* These tubes give origin to the tubes of Bellini, in whose interior the urine is secreted. The number of these tubes is enormous, but gradually decreases in consequence of these tubes uniting at acute angles two by two, until their number is reduced to two hundred, which form a sort of *triangular pyramid*, known under the name of *pyramid* or *cone of Malphighi.* There are about ten or fifteen of such cones in each kidney, with rounded apices termed *papillæ*, and converging towards the hilus of this organ. The papillæ, which are the excretory ducts of the Malpighian cones, are surrounded by short, membranous cups or *infundibula*, four or five of which are united into a common cup or *calyx*, which calices unite again in their turn to form the *pelvis* of the kidney. The pelvis terminates in the *ureter* which enters the cavity of the bladder.

The *supra-renal capsules* are two spongy, glandular organs of a yellowish-brown color, without excretory ducts. They are situated in the upper end of each kidney, which is covered by them as by a cup. Their object is as yet unknown.

II. The Ureters.

These are two cylindrical membranous canals conducting the urine from the pelvis of the kidney to the bladder. They pass from the pelvis of the kidney to the inferior and posterior portion of the bladder, which they enter, passing obliquely through its muscular and mucous coat. They are of the size of a goose-quill, but they are extremely dilatable, as is seen in various cases of retention of urine, in the passage of calculi from the kidneys, pressure occasioned by tumors, and difficult urination.

III. The Bladder.

This is the largest of all reservoirs in the human organism containing secretions. Its size varies with the age, sex, or habits of a person, or according to the disease with which the organ is affected. The female bladder is larger than the male, which is supposed to be owing to the circumstance, that the former is more liable to distention from the more frequent retentions of urine to which the female is exposed. But there is another reason why women void the urine less frequently than men; it is this, men drink more than women. As regards age, old people have a larger bladder than young persons; the former, owing to a blunted sensibility, do not feel the want of urinating as often as the latter, and hence they are enabled to retain the urine much longer than young people. This leads to an increased distention of the bladder. So far as habit has an influence on the size of the bladder, it may be said that the bladder of those who are in the habit of retaining their urine as long as possible, is larger than that of persons who discharge it frequently, as soon as the least desire to urinate is felt. Morbid conditions of the bladder may either occasion a considerable distention of this organ, as in retention of urine, or else an excessive contraction, so that not even a few drops of urine can be retained in the bladder. When the bladder is full, it can be distinctly felt above the symphysis pubis as high up as the navel. Only the upper and posterior portion of the bladder is covered by the peritoneum, so that only the lower portion of the organ can be cut into without injuring the peritoneal covering. Posteriorly, the bladder is bounded by the rectum in the male, and by the uterus in the female. To the lower surface of the bladder in the male are attached the seminal vesicles and the excretory ducts carrying the semen from the testicles to the vesicles. The superior extremity of the bladder is attached to the umbilicus by means of the *urachus*, a strong fibrous band arising from the obliteration of the umbilical vesicle, a canal that is found only in the fœtus.

The internal surface of the bladder shows numerous folds of the mucous membrane, which assume a smooth appearance when distended; moreover, we discover numerous muscular bundles, forming prominences or *trabecula*, and determining the contractile power of the bladder.

At the lower extremity of the bladder we see three orifices, those of the ureters and the opening of the bladder into the urethra. This portion of the bladder is termed the neck of the bladder.

The bladder is composed of three *coats*. The outer coat is a continuation of the peritoneum, and is, therefore, a serous sac covering the bladder only partially, as stated before; the middle or muscular coat is composed of longitudinal and circular muscular fibres, which cross each other. The third coat is a thin mucous membrane, which dips into the urethra. Besides these various parts, the bladder is furnished with numerous nerves and blood-vessels.

IV. The Urethra.

The urethra is the excretory canal of the bladder, and is solely formed of the cellular and mucous tissues of this organ.

The male urethra differing essentially from the female, they have to be described separately.

The male urethra is a canal of from six to eight inches long, and from two to three lines wide, but can be sufficiently dilated to admit of the passage of instruments of four lines in size in operations for stone in the bladder.

The urethra commences at the neck of the bladder, passes obliquely through the prostate gland forwards and downwards, takes a semi-lunar curve under the symphysis pubis, ascends forwards and upwards, and, from the root of the penis, courses onwards to the tip of the glans along the bottom of the furrow formed by the juxta-position of the corpora cavernosa. It is appropriately divided into three portions, 1st, the *prostatic portion*, which extends from the neck of the bladder to the outer edge of the prostatic gland, and which contains the so called *caput gallinaginis* or *verumontanum*, an oblong triangular fold of the mucous membrane; 2d, the *membranous* portion, about three-fourths of an inch in length, narrow, very little dilatable, and not surrounded by the prostate gland or the corpora cavernosa; 3d, the *cavernous portion* of the urethra, which is surrounded by the corpora cavernosa, and the lower part of which, forming an enlargement in consequence of its being enclosed by the corpora cavernosa, is termed the *bulbus* of the urethra. The lower wall of this portion of the urethra is somewhat depressed, on which account, the introduction of the catheter is frequently impeded, and, if conducted with undue force, occasioning the much dreaded perforations of the perinæum. When empty, the mucous membrane of the cavernous portion is arranged in folds, which accounts for its extreme dilatability. Previous to the urethra reaching its external orifice, the lower side of this canal expands into the so called *fossa navicularis*, in which the first phenomena of gonorrhœa develope themselves.

The *female urethra* is only one inch and a half in length, and has neither a prostatic portion, nor corpora cavernosa. Females are without the prostate gland. The female urethra is wider than the male; it can be dilated to six lines. This shortness and dilatability of the female urethra accounts, in some respects, for the less frequent occurrence of stone in females, and for the facility with which stone is taken from the female bladder without the operation of lithotomy. For the same reason it is much easier and much less dangerous to introduce the catheter into the female urethra.

The female urethra extends in the pelvic cavity downwards and forwards, forming a slightly convex curve, then courses along the mesian line of the anterior wall of the vagina, passes forwards under the symphysis pubis, between the crura of the clitoris, and ends between the labia minora, a few lines in front of, and above the orifice of the vagina.

The Urinary Secretion.

The blood is conducted to the kidneys by their arteries, and, after passing through a multitude of ramifications, arrives at the cortical substance, where it is first transformed into venous blood which the renal veins carry to the inferior vena cava, and afterwards into urine, which passes from the cortical substance into the tubes of Bellini of the medullary substance and oozes from the orifices of the papillæ, as may be distinctly seen by pressing upon the latter with the finger. From the papillæ the urine is received into the infundibula, the calices, and lastly into the pelvis of the kidney, whence, by its own weight, and by the movements of the diaphragm during respiration, it is pushed forward into the ureters, and finally collects in the bladder which expels its contents as often as the desire for it is felt.

The evacuations of the bladder take place in a similar manner as those of the bowels. Under the influence of the will the transverse fibres of the membranous portion of the urethra become relaxed, in consequence of which a similar relaxation takes place with the fibres of the sphincter vesicæ, and the orifice of the bladder is opened. Shortly after, the transverse muscular fibres of the bladder compress it from all sides; a similar compression is made by the longitudinal fibres from the apex to the fundus. These contractions which take place with great uniformity and regularity, and are assisted by the voluntary action of the abdominal muscles, drive the urine towards the orifice of the bladder, through which it passes into the urethra which is attached to the bladder like a moveable tube to a syringe, and, being a contracted and continuous canal of uniform dimensions, discharges the urine in a single, coherent stream.

The force with which the urine is expelled, is about equal to the force that would be required to burst the bladder, if the urine should be prevented, by some mechanical obstacle, from being expelled.

The immediate expulsion of the urine is effected by means of the muscular contractions of the bladder. But the contractions themselves are brought about by the action of the nerves, a great many of which are distributed over the walls, and more especially over the neck of the bladder; they proceed from the spinal marrow, and the absence or deficiency of this nervous action causes paralysis of the bladder and a consequent inability on the part of this organ to perform its contractions.

One of the principal causes which excites the muscular activity of the bladder, is the urine; it is the most natural and the most frequent cause of its contractions. It stimulates the walls of the bladder. According to the quantity and quality of the urine, its stimulating effects are more or less speedily perceived by the bladder. This depends likewise more or less upon the sensitiveness of the inner surfaces of the bladder, and upon the fact, whether one is in the habit of holding the urine as long as possible, or of voiding it as soon as the least desire for it is felt.

In young persons this sensitiveness is greater than in old age. The contractions of the bladder in the young are much more vigorous and rapid than in old people. In females the sensitiveness seems likewise less, for the reason, probably, that a feeling of modesty impels them to hold the urine as long as possible. Individuals who lead a sedentary life; literary men who, while their attention is riveted to scientific subjects, lose sight of the indications of t[illegible]dder, are enabled to hold the urine a long time on acco[illegible] diminished sensitiveness of the inner surfaces of this o[illegible]

The forcible retention of the urine in the bladder, co[illegible] to the natural desire of voiding it, may be productive of inc[illegible] culable mischief. The full bladder crowding upon the adjoining organs, a variety of distressing feelings are excited in consequence; stinging pains are experienced in the urethra, perinæum, and at the neck of the bladder; anxiety, palpitation of the heart, sweat, and even fainting fits are experienced, and the emission of the urine, if it is finally to be accomplished, becomes exceedingly difficult, or even a dangerous retention of urine sets in. It is said that the celebrated astronomer, *Tycho de Brahe*, perished at the table of Queen Christina of Sweden, in consequence of suppressing a natural desire of voiding the urine.

Foreign bodies in the bladder, such as stone, coagula, a piece of a probe, diseases of the prostate gland, hypertrophy of this organ, strictures of the urethra, spasms of the neck of the bladder, irritate this portion of the bladder, increase the sensitiveness and multiply the contractions of this organ. The same effect is produced by inflammation of the bladder, irritation of the bladder by foreign substances, which the urine derives from the circulatory fluid, by the internal and external use of Cantharides; such causes may occasion a continual desire to urinate, without a drop of urine being discharged.

The irritability of the bladder may be increased, and frequent contractions of this organ may be occasioned by various other diseases, such as painful hæmorrhoids, diseases of the rectum, cancer or polypus of the uterus, etc.

The rapidity of the flow of urine differs according to the age and constitution of the individual. In old people the flow is slower than in young persons. In stricture of the urethra the stream is frequently interrupted, and the discharge of the urine takes place drop by drop. If the stream rushes onward to a distance, we may regard this as a sign of strength.

The size of the stream depends upon the width of the urethra and upon its dilatability. In young persons the stream is larger than in old people. During an erection the stream is thinner, because the tension of the urethra prevents its full dilatation, and, besides, alters its course. If the prepuce covers the glans too tightly, the urine accumulates in the fossa navicularis, before being discharged.

Towards the close of an emission of urine, when the bladder is nearly emptied, the flow of urine slackens, and the stream stops, afterwards reappears more feebly and for a little while, again intermits and again makes its appearance. These last contractions of the bladder are performed partly by the muscular fibres of the bladder, partly by the muscles of the perinæum. The dribbling which takes place in some cases towards the end of the emission, which had been otherwise satisfactory as respects vigor and continuance, depends upon a deficiency of muscular action.

The urinary secretion of the female differs somewhat from that of the male. The female urethra being shorter, the stream which it discharges is less vigorous. The labia minora direct it downwards, and, in order to prevent the wetting the external pudendum and the thighs, females have to spread their lower limbs more than males during the act of micturition. The stream being moreover larger, females are able to accomplish it in a much shorter time than males. The greater width of the urethra may likewise be the cause of the more sudden and involuntary emission of urine in the case of females under the impulse of fright, fear, or in consequence of tickling, etc.

Physical Properties of the Urine.

The urine of the female contains more water and more saline particles than that of the male. In return the male generally secretes a larger quantity of urine than the female. Females are less subject to diseases of the urinary organs than males.

The urine which is secreted within twenty-four hours, weighs from three to five pounds. This quantity varies more or less according to the quantity of liquid that a person drinks in that period of time. Beverages which contain carbonic acid increase the secretion of urine; spirituous drinks diminish it. Various plants, and even nutrient vegetables, such as parsley, potatoes, beer, and such drugs as colchicum, digitalis, turpentine, saltpetre, bicarbonate of soda, cream of tartar, cantharides, etc., promote the secretion of urine by virtue of their specific action upon the kidneys. In the winter season, and in cold climates, more urine is secreted within twenty-four hours than in warm climates where the cutaneous exhalation is more abundant. This shows that the action of the skin and that of the kidneys are in alternate relation to each other. Children emit a large quantity of urine, which is pale and clear as water. Old people secrete a comparatively smaller quantity of urine, which is darker, and contains a good deal of urate and phosphate of lime.

In diseases, the secretion of urine may either be decreased or increased, or even entirely suppressed. In diabetes mellitus the urine is not only secreted in an excessive quantity, but it likewise contains a good deal of saccharine matter which may be obtained from the urine in the shape of crystals by evaporating the liquid. In diabetes insipidus, and in pulmonary phthisis, the urinary secretion is likewise increased; in fevers, in diseases of the liver and heart, and more particularly in dropsy, it is diminished, and in cholera and disorganizations of the kidney it is entirely suppressed.

The color of healthy urine is of a pale or orange yellow. In the morning the urine is generally darker, more saturated; this darker color is occasioned by the uroxanthin, a coloring matter of urine. In fevers, in diseases of the liver, in arthritis and rheumatism, etc., the urine frequently assumes a red-brown, dark-yellow, greenish, or some other color, and deposits a quantity of sediment. The normal chemical constituents of the urine are sometimes increased, at other times decreased in disease. In nervous diseases, in violent nervous pains, hysteria, megrim, the urine is generally pale and reacts less as an acid.

Several kinds of food and drugs modify the color of the urine. Beets, the fruit of the cactus opuntia, campeachy wood, Peruvian balsam, cochineal, madder, impart a reddish color to urine; rhubarb tinges it yellow; indigo and Prussian blue tinge it greenish and blue.

Urine, which is clear and transparent in health, is apt to become cloudy and turbid in disease. This cloudiness of the urine is partly owing to the anomalous chemical constituents of the urine, partly to the admixture of organic substances, such as: mucus, albumen, fat, blood, semen, pus, etc.

The odor of recently-voided urine is peculiarly aromatic, and not very disagreeable. After standing for a while, and cooling, it loses this odor, and assumes the characteristic smell of urine. Afterwards, according as the urine is more or less disposed to become decomposed, the smell changes to sour, and finally becomes ammoniacal and fetid.

In hysteria and other nervous affections, urine has no odor; in Bright's disease, which is generally accompanied with dropsy, and where the urine contains a good deal of albumen, it smells like broth; in diabetes mellitus it has at first an insipid smell which, after the sugar begins to ferment, changes to the odor of alcohol; in blennorrhœa of the bladder and in retention of urine, it has an offensive smell as soon as it is emitted.

The ordinary smell of urine is likewise altered by certain kinds of food or drugs. Asparagus, cabbage, cauliflower, impart a very unpleasant smell to urine; turpentine, rosin, balsam of copaiva or other kinds of balsam, give it the odor of violets; juniper berries, valerian, garlick, castoreum, musk, impart to the urine the odor which is peculiar to these substances.

A peculiar and not very frequent phenomenon is the *shining* of the urine. In one case this shining was observed in the winter-season immediately after the urine had been voided; it shone for half a minute like a fire-fly, after which the luminous appearance diminished. In another case the urine was observed to shine after it touched the wall or the soil; in some cases this phenomenon has been observed for two or three minutes in succession. This shining of the urine is a natural property of this fluid in the case of the civit-cat, the iltis, and other animals. This shining probably results from the presence of phosphorous nitrogen, arising from the deoxydation of phosphoric acid and carbon contained in the urine.

The chemical constituents of the urine in its normal or morbid state, and the various changes which this fluid undergoes, will not be described in this work, which was not designed to convey this sort of information.

The Sexual Organs.

These organs are similar, in their arrangement, to the urinary organs. Their destination is not, like that of the other viscera, to preserve the individual, but to propagate the species. Their constituent parts are: a gland which secretes the semen, and its excretory duct; a reservoir which receives and matures the semen, and a canal going to the surface of the body. The division of the sexual organs into external, middle and internal, is not applicable to both sexes; for that portion of the male organs, which corresponds to the internal female organs, is situated outside of the abdominal cavity. It would be more appropriate to class the sexual organs under two heads, *organs of generation* and *organs of fecundation;* the former prepare the seminal fluid, the latter perform the function of fecundation during the sexual act. The male organs of generation are *the testicles, spermatic duct* and *seminal vesicles;* the female organs are: the *ovaries, Fallopian tubes* and *uterus.* The male organs of fecundation are: the *penis;* and the female organs: the *vagina* and *vulva.*

I. The Male Sexual Organs.

The testicles, which secrete the semen, are the most essential portion of the organs of generation; they determine the sexual character of the man; their loss annihilates his generating faculty, and either renders nugatory, or effaces all his other sexual attributes. They are attached to the spermatic chords, and lie close together in the bottom of the scrotum, the right one a little higher than the left; they consist of the testicle properly speaking, and of the epidydimis.

The testicle has an ovoid, somewhat flattened shape. It is not quite perpendicular, its upper extremity being somewhat turned forwards and outwards, its lower extremity backwards and downwards, its anterior border somewhat downwards, and its posterior upwards.

The epidydimis is laid alongside the posterior border of the testis like a clasp; its larger, upper extremity is termed the globus major, and its thinner, lower extremity, which unites with the vas deferens, is termed the globus minor or cauda.

The testicle is surrounded by a fibrous membrane which determines the shape of the testicle, and, from its inner surface sends off a number of processes which dip into the substance of the testicle, and divide it into several hundred lobules, each of which is composed of several exceedingly convoluted seminiferous tubuli. These tubuli are about $\frac{1}{170}$ of an inch in diameter; they are united by cellular tissue and blood vessels, and constitute the parenchyma of the testicle. This parenchyma is very soft, and has the appearance of yellow or grey marrow deposited between the above-mentioned processes of the surrounding membrane. The marrow is composed of the seminiferous tubuli or ducts of which about 800 have been counted, and the united length of which amount to about 850 to 2500 feet.

II. The Seminal Ducts; or, Vasa Deferentia.

These are to the organs of generation what the ureters are to the bladder. Each vas deferens extends from the cauda of the epidydimis, of which it forms the continuation, to the seminal vesicle of the same side. At first it forms a convoluted duct, after which it passes upwards in a direct course along the posterior part of the spermatic cord, and along the spermatic canal to the internal abdominal ring. From the ring it is reflected inwards to the side of the fundus of the bladder, and descends along its posterior surface, crossing the direction of the ureter to the inner border of the vesicular seminalis, approaching that of the opposite side. It is through this open triangular space, where the bladder and the rectum meet, that the bladder has to be cut into from the perinæum in the operation of lithotomy. The vas deferens terminates at the base of the prostate gland by uniting with the duct of the vesicula seminalis, aad constituting the ejaculatory duct.

The structure of this canal is remarkable on account of the thickness of its parietes, which is so great that the canal can be easily felt in the spermatic cord.

III. The Spermatic Cord.

It is composed of arteries, veins, lymphatics, nerves, the excretory duct of the vesicle, and the investing tunics. It commences at the internal abdominal ring, where the vessels of which it is composed, converge, and passes obliquely along the spermatic canal; the cord then escapes at the external abdominal ring, and descends through the scrotum to the posterior border of the testicle. The left cord is somewhat longer than the right, and permits the left testicle to descend a little lower than the right. It is covered by a smooth fibrous membrane which it has in common with the external tunica vaginalis testis. This membrane extends through the inguinal canal down to the bottom of the scrotum, in the shape of a cylindrical bag which is enlarged below, and lines the spermatic cord and testicle of one side, without, however, forming a cavity; but, by its internal surface it adheres to the spermatic cord, and is united to the testicle by means of the tunica vaginalis. Externally the cord is surrounded by a thin muscular expansion capable of elevating the scrotum towards the abdominal ring.

IV. The Vesiculæ Seminales.

These are two lobulated and somewhat pyriform bodies situated on the under surface of the base of the bladder, and converging towards the base of the prostate gland. They are about two inches in length. Their upper surface is in contact with the base of the bladder; the under side rests on the rectum. Each vesicula is formed by the convolutions of a single tube, which gives off several irregular cœcal branches. It is enclosed in a dense fibrous membrane, and is constricted beneath the prostate gland into a small excretory duct. The vas deferens, somewhat enlarged and convoluted, lies along the inner border of each vesicula, and is included in its fibrous investment. It communicates with the duct of the vesicula, and forms the ejaculatory duct. This is about three quarters of an inch in length, and running forward, first between the base of the prostate and the isthmus, and then through the tissue of the verumontanum, opens upon the mucous membrane of the urethra, near its fellow of the opposite side, at the anterior extremity of that process.

V. The Prostate Gland.

This gland resembles a Spanish chesnut both in size and form. It surrounds the commencement of the urethra for a little more than an inch of its extent, and is situated upon the rectum, through which it may be felt with the finger. It consists of three lobes, two lateral and a middle lobe or isthmus, which are united together by a firm celular membrane that surrounds the whole gland. Its surface is smooth. The mucous membrane of the urethra being continuous with that of the excretory ducts of the gland, an inflammation of the urethra may spread onward to, and involve the gland.

VI. Cowper's Glands.

These are two small lobulated and somewhat compressed glands of the size of peas. They are situated in front of, and close behind the prostate gland, above the corpus spongiosum of the penis, to which they are attached by strong fibres. They consist of small lobules and vesicles, the excretory ducts of which unite into a larger duct three-fourths of an inch in length, and opening upon the lower surface of the urethra.

Their destination is scarcely any better known than that

of the prostate gland; and, on account of their small size, they are not of much practical importance.

VII. The Penis.

The penis is the medium of sexual union between the male and female. The urethra being the canal through which the male semen is discharged into the internal sexual organs of the female: it is one of the constituent parts of the male organs of generation. If the urethra had no other destination than merely to facilitate the escape of the urine from the bladder, a simple orifice at the surface of the body, as in the female, would be sufficient. Next to transmitting the semen, the penis discharges another very important mechanical function, viz: to excite the sexual tone in the female organs. This exultation of the female organs is an essential condition for the reception of the semen by the female. Hence the penis has to be so arranged as not only to be capable of erection but also of elongation. Otherwise it could not possibly exercise its sexual stimulation either by pressure or friction. The penis is provided with three dilatable bodies by means of which this purpose is accomplished. The entire penis is covered by the skin, and, at its root, is suspended to the mons veneris by a suspensary ligament. The skin is continuous with that of the mons veneris and scrotum, and with the skin of the adjoining parts. It is a thin skin, and is united to the subjacent parts by means of a loose cellular tissue which is capable of dilatation and extension. At the anterior extremity of the penis the skin is reflexed inwards as far as the fossa behind the glans; this reflexed portion of the skin changes to mucous membrane, and is reflexed back again over the glans. This anterior portion of the outer skin covering the glans is thinner, very delicate, and provided with a looser cellular tissue; it is termed the *foreskin* or prepuce, and generally covers, and even overhangs the tip of the glans, although it can be drawn back as far as the groove behind the glans. The prepuce is composed of the outer skin, and the subjacent mucous membrane; these two parts are separated by loose cellular tissue. In front, opposite the orifice of the urethra in the glans, the foreskin has a roundish slit of different size; the posterior half of the prepuce is composed of its inner layer, which is always more closely adhering and tighter than the outer skin or layer, and is united to the glans except in the middle, where it is attached by the frænulum to the urethra. On the inner side of the internal layer we have from two to three rows of follicular glands, which secrete a fatty, thick, strong-smelling substance of a white-yellow color, the abnormal accumulation of which, especially with a tight prepuce, sometimes occasions inflammatory symptoms, with small ulcers on the glans, *balannorrhœa*, which might be mistaken for syphilis by uninformed persons. If the prepuce is so long that it hangs beyond the glans like a tube, and if the foreskin is moreover so tight that it cannot be drawn back over the glans, we term this condition *phymosis*, which, in consequence of impurities accumulating behind the prepuce, or in consequence of an excessive secretion from the follicles, may lead to a painful inflammation of the mucous membrane, an inconvenience which Turks and Jews endeavor to prevent by circumcision. The *suspensory ligament* of the penis is composed of a bundle of strong fibres, of a triangular, flat shape, going from the symphysis pubis to the root of the penis.

The *corpora cavernosa* of the penis on its dorsum or sides, are composed of an exceedingly composite tissue of blood-vessels anastomosing with wide orifices; they are surrounded by a firm, fibrous membrane, sending processes into the tissue, by means of which it is divided into meshes within which the blood-vessels are embedded. There are two corpora cavernosa, one on the right, and the other on the left side, arising posteriorly by two roots from the inner borders of the ascending rami of the ischia. In front of the symphysis pubis both become enveloped in a fibrous covering, and, by a vertical, fibrous septum, are divided into two halves. Inferiorly, where they unite, a shallow furrow is formed, through which the urethra courses. The anterior extremity of the corpora cavernosa forms a truncated cone which is surrounded by the glans. Superiorly another furrow is formed, through which the dorsal vein of the penis, two arteries and nerves course. The distribution of the blood-vessels in the corpora cavernosa is different from that in other parts, and is principally calculated to admit of a speedy transmission of the fluid from the arteries into the veins. The *glans* forms the anterior extremity of the penis, and somewhat represents a truncated cone, the apex of which contains the orifice of the urethra. Behind the glans we discover a furrow, termed *corona glandis*. The surface of the glans is covered by a delicate mucous membrane, which is richly provided with follicles in the region of the corona. The tissue of the glans is spongy, erectile, like that of the corpora cavernosa. The glans seems to be a continuation and enlargement of the corpora cavernosa.

The Female Sexual Organs.

I. Ovaria.

The ovaria are to the female that which the testes are to the male: germ-preparing organs, and, therefore, the most essential portions of the organs of generation. Their shape and structure remind one of the testes, and, indeed, the ancients called them the female testes. They are two oval bodies, somewhat compressed from before backwards, and not quite as large as the testes. They are situate horizontally in the entrance of the small pelvis, in a fold of the broad ligaments, behind the Fallopian tubes, one on each side of the uterus. They are of a whitish color with a reddish tinge; previous to pubescence their surface is smooth, but after menstruation, conception or parturition, it becomes cracked. Immediately previous to the first menses their size is the largest; as the female advances in age, their size and shape becomes altered; they become thinner, harder, more elongated, and in old women they shrink up to one third of their original volume.

The ovaries are connected to the upper angles of the

uterus at each side by means of a rounded cord, the *ligament of the ovary*. By the opposite extremity they are connected by another and a shorter ligament to the fimbriated extremity of the Fallopian tube.

Each ovary is composed of a firm, whitish, shining fibrous covering which is intimately connected with the peritonæum; and of an internal substance composed of a number of blood-vessels and dense cellular tissue, the parenchyma of the ovary. This parenchyma contains from twelve to twenty perfectly closed membranous sacs, the *Graafian vesicles*, each of which is composed of three parts: 1, the *vesicle* properly speaking which is about three lines in diameter; its outer firm envelope adheres to the parenchyma, and its fluid interior contains a number of small granules which accumulate near the surface on the vesicle and constitute the *ovisacs* or receptacles of, 2, the human *ovum*, which is scarcely visible to the unarmed eye. The peripheral portion of the ovum is composed of *albumen*, the inner portion of the *yolk*, with numerous larger and smaller granules. In this yolk, but somewhat near the surface, we find 3, the sò-termed *germinal vesicle* discovered by Purkinge; it is transparent, rounded, surrounded by a very delicate envelope and containing in its interior a clear fluid, in which we observe through the microscope the *germinal spot* discovered by Wagner.

II. The Uterus.

This is a single hollow organ, in which the development of the fœtus takes place. It has an oblong, pyriform shape. Its broad, thick fundus is directed upwards, its flat, cylindrical neck downwards. The lowest portion of the neck projects forwards into the vagina, and is the *vaginal portion of the uterus*. The posterior surface of the body of the uterus is flatter than the posterior, and the *broad ligaments* are attached to the sides. The *round ligaments* are real prolongations of the substance of the womb, emanating from the sides of the fundus in the shape of rounded cords enclosed in the anterior layer of the broad ligaments, extend through the inguinal canal to the external pubic region, and are lost in the superficial fascia.

In proportion to the size of the organ, the cavity of the uterus is small; in females who have not yet borne children, the shape of this cavity resembles a triangle whose sides are bent inwards. The basis of the triangle corresponds to the fundus of the uterus. At the angles of the basis are the orifices of the Fallopian tubes. The summit of the triangle represents an elongated narrow canal with two openings, an upper one, *the interior orifice*, and a lower one, *the exterior orifice* of the womb. In virgins the exterior orifice is a transverse slit; but in females who had children, the orifice is rounded.

The substance of the uterus is composed of three layers. The outer layer, which is a duplicature of the peritonæum, is only seen on the fundus and body of the organ; the inner layer is a mucous membrane continuous with that of the Fallopian tubes, and forming within the neck of the uterus two or three longitudinal folds, from which smaller folds branch off on the sides, the whole of which resemble the stem and winged extremity of a feather, and are termed *arbor vitæ*. Between the little folds we perceive larger mucous glands which are very frequently of the shape of rounded, closed, prominent vesicles, and in this condition are termed *ovula of Naboth*. In the uterine cavity proper, the mucous membrane is without any folds and is dotted with small shaggy flocks and innumerable, tubular, perpendicular follicles acquiring a considerable development during pregnancy. The middle layer constitutes the hard genuine substance of the uterus.

The size, shape, position and condition of the uterine cavity undergo numerous modifications in the different ages of the female. The uterus of a young woman is two and a half inches long; it has a breadth of sixteen lines at the fundus, and of only nine lines at the neck. After parturition the uterus loses forever its virginal condition, and, on account of the relaxation of its ligaments, descends somewhat in the pelvic cavity. This likewise takes place transitorily during every monthly period.

The pressure which is exercised upon the adjoining organs by the impregnated uterus, accounts for the derangements of the alvine and urinary functions, the difficulty of breathing, the jaundice, the swelling and numbness of the feet, the distension and hardness of the abdomen, and the consequent tendency of carrying the upper part of the body backward.

The most remarkable changes of form take place in the neck and vaginal portion of the uterus. Having been once distended by pregnancy, the external orifice of the uterus never again assumes its flattened shape with the transverse split, but becomes rounded, with the lips standing apart, and the margins notched inconsequence of the lacerations which the external uterine orifice suffers during a first parturition, and which impart to it a cartilaginous consistence.

III. The Fallopian Tubes.

These tubes are given off from the upper portion of the uterus, and extend to the sides of the small pelvic cavity. They are five inches in length. Enclosed in the broad ligaments, they at first run in a straight line, and afterwards form an outward curve with fringed or fimbriated extremities, as if they had been bitten off. The fringes, when erect, form a funnel-shaped space, which embraces the ovary at the moment when an ovum escapes from a Graafian vesicle. The ovum passes through the tube into the uterus, in whose cavity it either disappears by absorption, or is changed to a fœtus. In rare cases it happens that the ovum remains within the tube, and is there transformed into a fœtus. This kind of pregnancy is termed Fallopian pregnancy, which always terminates unfavorably.

IV. The Vagina.

The vagina is a canal which leads from the uterus to the external pudendum and receives the penis during coït. It is dilatable and membranous, from five to six inches long, and fifteen to twenty lines wide, and situated between the bladder and rectum. Its course is slightly downwards and forwards, corresponding to the axis of the small pelvis in which it is imbedded. The upper extremity forms a circular cul-de-sac, embracing the neck of the uterus, and somewhat larger posteriorly; the anterior extremity forms a longitudinal split, terminating in the external pudendum. Its position between the rectum and bladder, and its proximity to the urethra, explains how one and the same cause may affect all these parts together; how, for instance, a violent and continued pressure of the head of the child during labor may cause a sloughing of these parts, and a consequent recto or vesico-vaginal fistula.

The walls of the vagina are about one line in thickness, dilatable and relaxed, and are composed of two closely interwoven membranes. The outer membrane is a firm *cellular membrane*, traversed by a numerous network of veins; the internal membrane is a delicate *mucosa*, continuous with that of the uterus and that of the labia minora. On the anterior wall of the vagina, this mucous membrane forms on both sides of a longitudinal sutsure numerous transverse rugæ, more particularly at the entrance of the vagina. These rugæ disappear more and more by coït and parturition. The mucous membrane is furnished with a multitude of follicles. Near the entrance the vagina is surrounded by circular muscular fibres, termed *constrictor vaginæ;* these fibres start from the lower side of the symphysis pubis, and coalesce with the constrictor ani. Numerous blood-vessels and nerves course along with the vagina.

V. The External Pudendum.

First, we notice the so called *mons veneris*, which is a prominence situated in front of the symphysis pubis, is composed of adipose cellular tissue, and covered with frizly hair.

The *labia majora* are two thick membranous folds, constituting the sides of the external pudendum. They communicate with the integuments of the mons veneris and those of the perinæum; at the posterior extremity, close to the entrance of the vagina, there is a small depression, termed the *fossa navicularis.* Externally the labia majora consist of a delicate, rather hairy skin, continuous with that of the thighs and pubic region; the inside covering resembles a mucous membrane, is thin and smooth, reddish in young, and pale in old age. Both the outer and inner sides enclose a loose adipose cellular tissue and a number of mucous follicles opening on the inner side. In the virgin both lips are closely united, forming a longitudinal slit; after frequent coït and parturition, they remain permanently separated more or less by the labia minora, which protrude between the former.

The *labia minora* or *nymphæ*, likewise constitute two membranous folds, emanating from the labia majora. Posteriorly they are closer together than anteriorly; externally they terminate in a cock's-comb-shaped, indented, free margin. They consist of a delicate, red mucous membrane, richly provided with nerves, and hiding between its external and internal layers a loose cellular tissue and a number of mucous glands. At the anterior and superior extremity, each lip divides into two crura, the lower ones of which unite with the clitoris, and and the upper ones of which, above the clitoris, coalesce, forming a sort of cap or prepuce.

It is only in females in whom they do not protrude, that the labia minora have the rosy color of a mucous membrane; if protruding, they become drier, harder, assume a brown color, and, if the sexual organs are abused, they sometimes become so relaxed that they hang down like flaps of an inch in width. Among the women of the Hottentots and Bosjemans, they are from six to eight inches long, and have been described by travellers as aprons. Among certain tribes of northern Africa, they are habitually so long that they have to be cut off.

The *clitoris* is a body that resembles the male penis. It consists of two corpora cavernosa, has a glans, prepuce and double frænulum, but no meatus urinarius. The clitoris is situated below the anterior commissure of the labia minora, and is covered by the prepuce. It arises by two crura from the ascending rami of the ischia, to each of which an erector muscle is attached; the corpora cavernosa unite under the symphysis pubis, terminating in the glans of the clitoris which reaches beyond the prepuce in the shape of a roundish body of the size of a pea. Superiorly the clitoris is united to the symphisis pubis by means of a frænulum, and inferiorly to the labia minora by means of another frænulum.

This portion of the pudendum is richly endowed with nerves and vessels, and is the principal seat of the thrill during coït.

In the southern climate the clitoris is larger than in the temperate and frigid zones. Among the women of Abyssinia, among the Mendingas and Ibbos, its size is so considerable that it is a popular usage to clip off a part of it. When, after the conversion of the Abyssinians to Christianity, the circumcision of the women was abolished as a remnant of paganism, the men rebelled against this innovation, and the opposition was not appeased until a surgeon was sent by the propaganda from Rome, who declared the restoration of the former custom necessary.

Among our own women the clitoris is sometimes so large that a belief in the existence of hermaphrodites has been suggested by this abnormal size; that is to say, female sexual organs with a male penis, a malformation which has induced an unnatural satisfaction of the sexual instinct between two women. In the case of a woman of thirty-five years, the clitoris had the size of the penis of a boy of two years, and was capable of erection and abnormal sexual satisfaction; in another case the clitoris had the ordinary thickness, but four times its natural length; all the other characters of the female pudendum were preserved in their natural form. In this case the clitoris was an hindrance to sexual intercourse, and was amputated with success.

The triangular space between the clitoris, meatus urinarius, and labia minora, is termed the *vestibule* of the vagina.

The meatus urinarius forms a small, pad-shaped ring, and is situated below the clitoris and above the entrance to the vagina.

In virgins, the greater portion of the *vaginal orifice* which is covered by the labia, is closed by the *hymen.* This hymen consists of two folds of the mucous membrance, and has various shapes; generally it is semi-lunar, with a concave margin. Sometimes it is circular, covering the whole orifice, with a perforation in the centre. Very seldom the vagina is closed entirely, which would prevent the discharge of the menstrual blood. Generally the hymen is torn during the first sexual embrace, and its remnants are termed the *myrtle-shaped warts.* In some cases, however, the hymen remains intact after repeated intercourse, and I myself have been obliged in the case of a primipara, to separate the hymen with the knife during the act of parturition.

Physiology of the Sexual Functions.

The highest object of the sexual functions is the propagation of the species. This is effected by the sexual act and consequent fecundation.

I. The Sexual Act.

The object of the sexual act on the part of man is, to discharge the semen into the sexual organs of the female, and on the part of woman to receive the seminal fluid. The sexual delight which precedes the act, increases in proportion as the contact of the sexual organs becomes more intimate. By merely touching the mammæ, both the mammæ and the penis sometimes become erect, the woman experiences shooting stitches in the mammæ and abdomen, palpitation of the heart, trembling, chills; excitable or debilitated females are even seized with convulsions. The penis and the tissue of the clitoris become erect, and the constrictor muscle of the vagina dilates its orifice and changes it to a rounded opening. On inserting the penis into the vagina, the nerves of the clitoris are first touched by the glans, and the sexual delight is increased; passing onward under the clitoris, the glans penetrates with some difficulty between the prominences of the vestibule, the dorsum of the penis comes in contact with the glans of clitoris, and the whole space of the vagina is filled up by the penis.

In virgins the sexual delight is increased even by the pain which the tearing of the hymen causes; the narrowness and the pleasant temperature of the vagina, its prominences here and there, and the rhythmical contractions of the constrictor vaginæ, facilitate the delightful friction of the penis; the voluntary movements of the penis, and the involuntary action of the erector muscles, increase the excitement to the highest degree, which terminates in the male with the emission of the semen, and in the female after the penis had been withdrawn from the vagina, or the penis has become relaxed. By means of the vaginal friction, the orifice of the womb may possibly be opened so that the semen is enabled to reach the interior of the womb, but in most cases it flows back again out of the vagina.

The emission takes place involuntarily by the contraction of the ejector muscles; after the emission is terminated the stimulation of the nervous tissues generally ceases, as well as the afflux of blood to the arteries of the penis; the blood again flows backwards through the veins, and the penis becomes relaxed. The erection of the clitoris likewise ceases.

This sexual orgasm is frequently succeeded by languor, drowsiness, sadness, irritable mood; hence the proverb: "*omne animal post coïtum triste*," after coït every animal feels out of humor.

II. Fecundation.

In order that fecundation or conception may take place, it is necessary that the ovum should actually be touched by the semen, and not merely by the seminal aura; and, secondly, that the semen should contain a sufficient number of spermatozoa. We will now proceed to consider these elements and laws of conception more in detail.

The Male Semen.

On coming out of the urethra, the male semen consists of a thin fluid which is soon succeeded by a fluid of more consistence, and forms a mixture of the secretions of the testicles, spermatic ducts, seminal vesicles, Cowper's glands, of the prostatic fluid, and probably of the mucus of the urethra. As was said above, the semen consists of a thin milky, and of a thick, viscid and albuminous portion. If the semen is exposed to the air, the fluidity of these elements increases, and a more intimate commingling takes place. The semen spreads a peculiar odor, has an alkaline reaction; its chemical constituents are water, mucus, albumen, natrum, phosphate and muriate of lime, phosphorus, and a peculiar animal substance, termed *spermatine*. If the semen is seen through the microscope, we discover floating in it small filiform bodies which have been termed *spermatozoa*. They exist in every kind of animal semen, and are so characteristically shaped, that their presence is a sure indication of the character of the fluid. In the spermatozoa of the human semen, one extremity is large, *the head*, to which is attached a thread-shaped prolongation, *the tail;* their length is from $\frac{1}{30}$ to $\frac{1}{40}$ of a line.

If magnified to three or four hundred times their original size, in the recent semen, they move about very briskly in every direction; they agitate their tails, and even avoid small obstacles in their course. Gradually their movements become slower, and finally cease altogether. The duration and liveliness of these movements depend upon the strength of the individual from whom the semen came. The strength or debility of these spermatozoa indicates a higher or lower degree of fecundating power. They first show themselves at the age of pubescence, and probably disappear again with the complete extinction of the sexual power. Their complete absence indicates an inability on the part of man to fecundate the female ovum.

The Female Ovum.

The ovaries, the artificial removal or the destruction of which by disease is just as surely followed by sterility as the removal of the testicles in the male, contain from 12 to 20 ovula which we have described previously. In little girls the ovaries are very small and light, but towards the period of pubescence they increase rapidly in size and weight; at the critical period termed the period of involution, when the menstrual flow ceases, they, together with the ovula, disappear. Each menstrual period is characterized by an increased determination of blood towards the ovaries, which is particularly perceptible round the ovum that has reached the highest degree of maturity and which then reddens, swells and escape from its capsule. This little ovum is seized by the fimbriated extremity of the Fallopian tube and conducted to the uterus whence it escapes with the menstrual blood. After the escape of the ovum the ruptured vesicle becomes cicatrised, and forms a yellowish spot which Wagner terms the *germinal* spot. Formerly when the physiology of the female functions was yet little understood, it was supposed that this yellow spot was a sign of previous fecundation; but this spot is seen in girls who had never conceived; for a little ovum is detached at each menstruation, and after its escape, leaves this yellow spot.

The first menses generally make their appearance towards the fourteenth year, and the menstrual discharge ceases again between the forty-fifth and fiftieth year. It is a most important function in the female organism; irregularities as to time and quantity induce a variety of disturbances. The menstrual blood is dark and does not readily coagulate; during its discharge the mucous membrane of the uterus is renovated.

Before we pass to an examination of the difficult and interesting question, *how* and *where* the semen comes in contact with the ovum, it may not be out of place to describe the interesting experiments of artificial fecundation of the eggs of frogs that have been instituted by *Spallanzani*, *Prevost* and *Dumas*. Spallanzani watched the fecundating process as carried on by frogs in and out of the water. At the instant when the female wants to lay her eggs, the male spirts a clear fluid upon them, by which means fecundation takes place. Having covered the legs of the male with oil-silk, the eggs remained unfecundated, and a sufficient quantity of the fluid was found adhering to the oil-silk leggins, to enable him to collect some of it by means of a fine painter's brush. Every egg which he touched with this fluid, became fecundated. This experiment was repeated by Prevost and Dumas, and it was found that this direct fecundation was always accompanied by the presence of spermatozoa. This fact puts an end to the formerly prevailing opinion that fecundation was effected by a *seminal aura*. Semen and ova have been placed so near to each other, that the latter had to be touched by the seminal exhalation; but no fecundation took place, and was, on the other hand, effected immediately as soon as actual contact between the seminal fluid and the ovum had taken place. If the spermatozoa are motionless, consequently dead; or if they are sickly, or imperfectly developed, in such a case they are of no use as fecundating agents, and, if this should be the condition of the human spermatozoa, the male semen is unfit to carry on the process of fecundation, and sterility ensues.

Let us now enquire where the process of fecundation takes place in the human subject. Numerous experiments and investigations have recently shown that it is in the ovaries that the semen comes in contact with the ovum and that the first germ of the future man is formed. It is only among the inferior animals that the eggs are detached from their original abode previous to fecundation; among the higher species the male semen goes to the ovum while yet lodged in the ovary. On this account fecundation is most readily effected shortly previous to the menstrual period; for the ovum may have escaped from its vesicle, and is perhaps on its way to the uterine cavity, meeting the semen half way. Starting from this supposition it has been laid down as a rule that, in order to avoid fecundation, no intercourse with the female should be had eight days before, nor eight days after the menstrual period.

The supposition that the fecundating process takes place in the ovary, is fortified by the following reasons: 1. If animals are killed shortly after conception, semen is found in the ovaries; 2. The eggs of birds only reach the period of maturity gradually, and the ova of mammalia do not penetrate the uterine cavity until some time after the accomplishment of the sexual act, when the semen could no longer be fresh and possessed of fecundating power; 3. Pregnancy may take place beyond the uterine cavity; 4. If shortly after the sexual act the Fallopian tubes are tied, no fecundation takes place.

Formerly the process of fecundation was accounted for in a different manner. The doctrine was, that a seminal aura penetrated through the uterine cavity and the Fallopian tubes to the ovaries, where it effected the process of fecundation. This being accomplished, the fecundated ovum was conveyed into the uterine cavity for the purpose of further development. This opinion was undoubtedly very ingenious, but erroneous. Fecundation is only effected when both the male and female seminal secretions meet at one and the same moment. But this can only be accomplished when the semen is healthy, and the penis sufficiently erect to introduce the semen into the uterus. If the ovum is not sufficiently developed, if the tubes are closed, if the neck of the uterus is either closed or deviating from its normal axis, if the vagina is obstructed, etc., fecundation is impossible.

From these facts which have been abundantly established by modern physiologists, we infer that *the procreation of a new human being requires as a necessary condition the immediate contact of the semen and the ovum.*

The next question is, to ascertain *what part the semen and the ovum respectively take in the act of fecundation.*

To solve this question, a multitude of hypotheses have been resorted to. It was supposed that the semen of the male being composed of all the constituent parts of the body, it furnished the first elements towards the formation of the different organs and tissues of the new being. Or it was believed that the semen itself, together with the spermatozoa, after undergoing a number of transformations, formed the new man, or, at any rate, the principal portion of this new man, namely, the nervous system. Another opinion was, that the semen was a living fluid, and that it excited life and developments in a female germ, the ovum.

In regard to the product of the ovary, opinions were equally diversified. Some said that a vesicle was filled with semen which, like the semen of the male, consisted of the original elements of the various constituent organs of the body; others taught that the ovum was transformed into a receptacle for the spermatozoa to which it furnished sustenance; some again supposed that some unorganized substance that had the properties of gelatine, was the cause of life by exciting motion. Finally, according to the opinion of modern physiologists, such as *Valentin*, *Joh. Mueller*, *Wagner*, *Bischoff*, *Brûcke*, etc., *the ovum, after being detached from the ovary, derives from the semen the property of developing itself further in the uterus, and evolving a new being endowed with life, and resembling both the father and the mother.*

If a perfect commingling of the seminal secretions takes place, it is just as impossible for either the male or female to prevent conception, as it is otherwise impossible to determine the physical or moral qualities of the fœtus. Some of the ancients, physiologists and physicians, among whom we distinguish, *Anaxagoras*, *Aristoteles*, *Hippocrates*, fancied that the right testicle and ovary furnished the elementary constituents of the boy, and the corresponding left organs those of the girl. If this were so, it must certainly be possible, during intercourse, to cause either the left or right organs to be principally active; but this seems impossible so far as we know. But the opinion itself is erroneous; for we know of men who, after losing one testicle, procreated both male and female children; and so in regard to women: with one ovary only, boys and girls indifferently were the result of conception. Similar results were experimentally obtained in the case of rabbits.

It is likewise beyond the power of the male or female to determine by volition the number of ova that are to be fecundated. In the case of man, one ovum is the rule; but there are cases where two, three, and even four and five children were born at one birth.

Nevertheless, the physical and moral qualities of the fetal child are not entirely beyond the reach of the parents' influence. Such an influence is however exercised only gradually. The condition of the fœtus depends upon the moral state of the parents during the sexual act, and upon a certain degree of activity which is required to secure the proper performance of the act. It is past all doubt that the vitality of the child is more or less proportionate to the vigor and cheerfulness, or to the indifference and unwillingness which were displayed during coït. Excessive sexual intercourse results in the procreation of weakly children, whereas healthy and vigorous children are the consequences of a moderate and rational enjoyment of the sexual pleasure. Too frequent coït, excessive sexual passion, and even premature marriage, are prejudicial to child-bearing. To secure the highest degree of fecundity, the husband should be about ten years older than the wife. The fecundity of the human female is greatest up to the age of twenty-six years, that of the human male up to thirty-three. An active mode of life and bodily exercise favor conception, even among those who are obliged to live poorly, although want and starvation diminish the number of births proportionally to the high price of food. In warm climates and along the coast, conception takes place more readily than in colder climates. Some nations are distinguished in this respect. The fecundity of the Jewish females was known even to the Egyptians; negro women conceive more readily than white women; the Slavish race is, in this respect, superior to the Germanic nations. There are years when the number of births is much less than in others.

After an earthquake it was observed that for two years the women ceased to bear children.* After a war or an epidemic disease the number of births is generally much greater than ordinarily.

Conception generally takes place when the semen is retained after coït. However, this is not by any means a rule. Some women can tell immediately after the act whether conception has taken place; others know it only some days after by a series of peculiar sensations, such as vertigo, nausea, vomiting, colic, aversion to certain kinds of food and to sexual intercourse.

Conception depends upon both external and internal circumstances. The greatest number of pregnancies generally occurs during the months of May and June. Ardent women are said to conceive more readily in winter, colder women in summer. Indifference or aversion to intercourse is an obstacle to conception, although it has happened that women have conceived during sleep, and even after rape.

* This might have been the result of fright.—Ed.

SECTION II.

OF THE DISEASES OF THE SEXUAL AND URINARY ORGANS.

In the preceding section the anatomy and physiology of the urinary and sexual organs have been explained. We have seen that these organs perform exceedingly important functions in the human organism, and that the urinary organs in particular are necessary to the preservation of life and health, for they eliminate all such constituents of the blood as are no longer serviceable to the reproduction of the tissues, and which, if retained in the blood, would cause disease; hence we infer that the preservation and healthful condition of these organs are essentially necessary to the normal condition of the organism. We have likewise seen that the sexual organs subserve the purpose of procreation, and that their high object can only be accomplished by preserving them in health and strength, and enabling them to perform their peculiar process of secretion readily and without the least hindrance.

In the following sections we intend to describe and explain the various disturbances to which the functions of these organs are liable, and to indicate the remedies which are capable of restoring them to a state of health in the *quickest*, *safest*, *pleasantest* and most *lasting* manner. We shall likewise point out to the reader the rules and principles by the observance of which a derangement of their functions may be avoided.

We shall have to examine the diseases of these organs in a twofold point of view. Some of these diseases arise from causes which are of a general character and have nothing to do with syphilitic contagion; but by far the larger number is the result of syphilitic infection which is communicated by one sex to the other during the sexual act, and by which the highest earthly delight is not only converted into a source of loathsome and distressing disease, but which likewise results in the procreation of an unhealthy, miserable offspring. We will begin our work with the treatment of the more important class, the syphilitic diseases, premising a short indication of their probable origin and their successive development in the different periods of the world's history.

The first historical investigations of this disease were instituted from religious motives. Venereal diseases were represented as a punishment from God for sexual transgressions. At a later period, these investigations assumed a political character, and served to gratify national antipathies. The French termed the syphilitic disease "*mal de Naples,*" the Italians "*mal Francese,*" the Germans "*Franzosen.*" Oviedo, a Spaniard, derived the disease from the American Indians, as if to palliate the cruelties which had been perpetrated by his countrymen against the aborigines of America.

Science is interested in these historical investigations of the origin and spreading of the disease; for a knowledge of these facts may facilitate the treatment, and suggest correct views concerning the infectious character of the malady. Let us therefore cast a glance at its history.

The history of syphilis may be divided into three periods; the first extends to the end of the fifteenth century, or the epidemic of 1495; the second extends from this period to the time when Fernel made the discovery that syphilis is a specific poison; and the third period extends to the present day.

It is an established fact that the origin of the venereal disease is lost in the remotest antiquity. It seems superfluous to repeat in this place the various contradictory opinions in reference to this matter. The first allusions to venereal discharges are contained in the books of Moses. As regards genuine syphilis, it is not by any means impossible that this disease, like glanders and small pox, may have been transmitted to man by the brute creation. It is well known that many diseases are ingrafted upon the human species by animals, and are afterwards developed among mankind as a disease peculiar to them. It is not therefore, improbable that syphilis has a similar origin, which is somewhat confirmed by the derivation of the term syphilis from the Greek words, *sys*, swine, and *phileo*, to love.

Besides the allusions to a contagious discharge from the urethra, contained in the books of Moses, we find similar allusions in the writings of the ancient Greek physicians, from which the existence of syphilis may be inferred. Hippocrates mentions ulcers of the sexual organs, pustules of the penis, and a considerable number of other affections arising from the progressive development of syphilis.

Celsus describes every variety of chancre with or without phimosis, the indurated Hunterian chancre, and the phagedenic chancre.

Galen describes a case of gonorrhœa contracted by coït. Avicenna gave a detailed account of ulcers of the penis which resemble perfectly the modern chancre. Michael Scott relates cases of disease which were communicated to men by unclean females and vice vérsa, and which produced symptoms which resembled exactly the modern constitutional syphilis.

W. Saliceto, Lanfranc and their disciples describe ichorous, virulent or so-called acrid discharges inducing a variety of affections of the sexual organs and genuine buboes. A detailed account of syphilis is also found in the work of W. Becket who communicates the rules laid down for the prostitutes of the city of Winchester, according to which every diseased woman, if caught in the exercise of her trade, was fined one hundred shillings. These facts go to show that ancient authors were as well acquainted with syphilis as with the other maladies which they describe; only they did not know that the syphilitic disease was derived from a specific poison. They were unacquainted with the mode in which the poison was communicated, and they were particularly unacquainted with the constitutional consequences of primary syphilis. With the elder physicians constitutional syphilis was a form of lepra. Syphilis existed in the earliest ages, but its character was not yet known.

In 1494 the epidemic broke out. Some twenty different nations were invaded by it. In Germany the disease had been unknown previous to this time. The morals of the people were rigid, and prostitution was rare. Morever, there was little intercourse between the different German states. This was different in other countries, especially in Italy: a wide-spread commerce on the sea, luxurious living, shameless immorality, and the celibacy of the priests naturally spread the disease far and wide.

The campaign of Charles VIII. of France was one of the chief causes of the spread of the epidemic; hence its name *morbus gallicus*, or French disease. In the month of August, 1494, Charles invaded Italy with a well appointed army, for the purpose of chastising Pope Alexander VI. who was opposed to his pretensions, and of conquering the kingdom of Naples, which had fallen to him as an inheritance. The soldiers carried off an immense booty, but at the same time the syphilitic disease. They termed it *souvenir* or *mal de Naples*, in which city it had existed previous to the arrival of the French, and where it exercised the greatest ravages among them. The assertion that the disease was brought by the Spaniards from America, is without any foundation; for it was first in 1495 that a Spanish army was sent to Italy, consequently one year after the character of the disease had already been established.

In Germany the spread of the disease was principally attributed to the lansquenets, a military rabble, who were constantly ready to sell their life and blood to the highest bidder. With what frightful rapidity syphilis spread in an army, was sufficiently demonstrated in the last wars. It was not to be wondered that syphilis should have spread throughout Europe in the fifteenth century, when the whole continent was traversed by military hosts; nor that physicians should have begun to suspect the connection between primary and secondary syphilis. One reason why this knowledge was so tardily obtained, was the fact that physicians were ashamed of treating ulcers of the sexual organs, and left this dirty business to quacks of every description.

The same confusion which prevailed as respects the origin of syphilis, likewise prevailed in regard to the mode in which the disease was transmitted. It was believed that the disease might be transmitted by the atmosphere, and that it might be introduced into and carried out of a convent through the lattice-door in the parlor. Fallopius fancied that the disease might be communicated by the holy water into which a syphilitic patient had dipped his finger. Only an obscure idea was had of the syphilitic poison.

It was not until the year 1556 that Fernel showed that the syphilitic disease originated in some specific cause emanating from some affected individual, and acting upon one in health. He deserves the credit of having opposed the opinion that the disease was communicated by the atmosphere. Forsaking the belief in astrological, cosmic or teleological ideas, which prevailed in his time, he succeeded in describing with great correctness the mode of transmission of the syphilitic disease. He teaches that it is contagious, and that contagion is indispensable to its transmission. Contagion cannot take place without actual contact, and the most frequent contact is during sexual intercourse. With a master's hand Fernel describes the symptoms by which the contagion is recognised, likewise the secondary or constitutional symptoms. Even after a lapse of three hundred years, Fernel's picture of the syphilitic disease is still true, and the recent additions have only served to make it appear still more so.

Fernel's' doctrines were perfected and confirmed by John Hunter and Carmichael, but the most scientific works on syphilis, in which the disease is discussed with all the light which modern science has shed upon every form of knowledge, emanate from the pen of Ricord of Paris, Simon of Hamburg, Sigmund of Vienna, Waller of Prague, etc.

First Series of Syphilitic Diseases.

It is peculiar to these diseases to arise either directly or indirectly from an impure coït, and to be transmitted to other persons by some specific contagion, somewhat in a similar manner to the inoculation of the small-pox. Hence it is that these diseases first break out on the sexual organs, and, by means of the lymphatic system, are thence carried through the whole organism. Generally the chancre either breaks out on the integuments of the penis, where the skin had been excoriated, or in some part where the delicate epidermis had been injured, as on the glans penis, on the mucous membrane of the pudendum, on the labia, etc.

We will distinguish this larger group of diseases into two divisions, 1st, *simple venereal diseases*, and 2d, *venereal or syphilitic diseases properly speaking*.

I. Simple Venereal Diseases.

These are diseases which have not the specific syphilitic character, and do not induce constitutional syphilis by penetrating the general organism. Among these diseases we number gonorrhœa and blennorrhœa, together with all the accessory and secondary affections belonging to these discharges, female gonorrhœa and common leucorrhœa.

II. Gonorrhœa of the Male.

By gonorrhœa we understand a violent inflammation of the mucous membrane of the urethra, with a discharge of purulent mucus.

The course of this disease is generally as follows:—From two to five days after an impure coït, the patients generally experience a peculiar itching at the tip of the penis, which, during an erection, increases to a real pain. This pain is aggravated during an emission of urine. In two or three days more, the orifice of the urethra becomes red, swollen and moist. Frequently a tension and drawing are experienced at this period in the spermatic cord, the testes, the inguinal region. After urinating, a slight burning pain is experienced, which increases from day to day. The swelling and redness of the urethra likewise increases, and a discharge, which is at first inconsiderable and is generally clear and viscid, takes place from the urethra, and causes the sides of the orifice to adhere. The linen looks stained, the glans swells more or less, becomes hot, red, and is painful during a walk. The erections are distressing, and are particularly frequent at night, disturbing sleep. On the eighth day, and sometimes earlier, the discharge increases, becomes thicker, of a yellowish-white color, milky. The inflammatory symptoms gradually increase in violence and extent. The pain during urination and during erections, reaches the highest degree of violence, and is no longer confined to the forepart of the penis, but extends over the whole organ. On account of the inflammation, the urethra becomes contracted; hence the stream of urine is no longer full and large, but divided. The discharge assumes a greenish-yellow tint, becomes thick, profuse, and has a peculiar, disagreeable odor. When sitting the patient experiences pain, and the perinæum even is sometimes swollen in consequence of the inflammation of Cowper's glands.

This second stage of gonorrhœa generally commences on the seventh or eighth day, and continues for eight days or a fortnight. It is of great importance in the treatment of the disease, that the first and second stages should not be confounded.

In the stage of decrease the first sign of improvement is, that the emission of urine and the erections are less painful, and finally become altogether painless; only the discharge continues, and changes to a whitish, viscid, thready secretion. The redness at the orifice of the urethra, and the swelling of the glans disappear. If these symptoms should continue for awhile, without being accompanied by pain, we term them secondary gonorrhœa or gleet.

Whatever cause is capable of inducing an inflammation of

the urethra, may likewise cause a gonorrhœal discharge. This need not necessarily be the result of an impure coït. New wine, unfermented beer, stimulating spices, a cold, exposure of the organs to the wind while urinating, frequently cause a gonorrhœal discharge which runs the same course as, and is similar to, genuine gonorrhœa.

As regards the disposition to gonorrhœa, it generally occurs among young people. Persons with a long and narrow prepuce are more easily infected than those whose prepuce glides loosely over the glans, or in whom the glans is not at all covered by this organ. In such cases the glans is much less sensitive, and hence less liable to the action of the gonorrhœal poison. Among the nations where circumcision is practised, gonorrhœa is much less frequent than among us.

A gonorrhœal discharge may likewise be induced by *mechanical or chemical causes*, by a *natural predisposition, climate, a peculiar structure of the sexual organs, and by constitutional debility.*

Among the *mechanical causes* of gonorrhœa, we may mention the introduction of the catheter or of a bougie into the urethra, mechanical injuries of the mucous membrane of this canal, calculi or other foreign bodies in the urethra, etc.

Among the *chemical causes* we note injections of irritating substances, abuse of spirits, spices, salt food, asparagus and beer.

As regards *predisposition*, persons of a plethoric habit, with blond hair, a fine white color, and a delicate frame, are more easily tainted than those who do not possess these qualities.

In regard to *climate*, it may be stated, that gonorrhœa occurs more frequently in a warm than in a cold climate.

So far as the *structure of the organs* is concerned, a large penis, a wide urethra lined with a thick mucous membrane, repeated infections, strictures, or disorganizations of the mucous tissue, facilitate the gonorrhœal contagion.

The forms of constitutional irritation which predispose one more particularly to gonorrhœa, are *cutaneous eruptions*, *scrofula*, *tubercles*, *gout*, *rheumatism* and *piles*. Onanism and venereal excesses may likewise cause a discharge from the urethra without any other infectious contact.

The most frequent cause of gonorrhœa is an *impure coït*. Even if the coït was not completed, and the penis was simply brought in contact with a diseased pudendum, infection may take place. It must not be imagined, however, that a specific or so termed virulent discharge is indispensable to effect this result. A gonorrhœal discharge may be induced by excessive sexual intercourse, even among married persons, by an imperfectly executed or an excessively prolonged coït; by having intercourse during the menstrual period, or during the last months of pregnancy, when the ordinary vaginal discharge becomes quite considerable, and sometimes very acrid, or by ulceration of the neck of the womb.

It is a remarkable fact, that some men can have sexual intercourse with women who have the whites, without being affected by this discharge, whereas other men are at once infected by these same persons. This must be owing to the fact, that some men are not susceptible to this kind of infection, whereas others are so to an extraordinary degree. I have known cases, and other authors have had a similar experience, that several men in succession had intercourse with the same girl, and that some of them were infected, others, on the contrary, remained intact. There are likewise cases where a gonorrhœal discharge took place without the least symptom of discharge or ulceration being perceptible in the girl, even after the strictest examination by a physician.

It may likewise happen that women had been infected by a man, and that previous to any discharge having yet made its appearance, they communicated the disease to the next customer.

A gonorrhœa which had developed itself after intercourse with a perfectly healthy woman, is frequently more obstinate, and more unyielding to treatment than a genuine syphilitic discharge. It is therefore necessary to be acquainted with the rules, by the observance of which a gonorrhœal infection can be prevented.

To this end every unnatural excitement should be avoided, before and during an embrace. Stimulation by means of spices or spirits, unnatural means of producing sexual excitement during the act, excessive enjoyment of the sexual pleasure, etc., are sometimes sufficient to excite a gonorrhœal discharge.

It is an established fact that the preservation of a man's health, especially in the full vigor of manhood, requires the enjoyment of sexual intercourse. Complete abstinence from all intercourse is sometimes followed by dangerous diseases, especially in healthy and vigorous men. Considering that there are many men in large cities, who do not get married because they either have not the means of supporting a family, or because they do not find any one whom they desire to marry, prostitutes seem to be a necessary evil for the time being. The following rules should be observed during sexual intercourse with a prostitute: the act should be accomplished in as short a time as possible, and, immediately after the ejaculation of the semen, the penis should be withdrawn, because it is a well-known fact that the susceptibility of the organ to the reception of the contagion is much increased.

After the coït the penis should at once be washed with a solution of soap, and the urine should be voided, because by this means the morbid matter which might have adhered to the parts, would again be easily expelled.

Some grease the penis with a fatty substance previous to its introduction into the vagina; by this means the pores of the skin are obstructed, and the poison is prevented from penetrating into the parts. The safest preventive is undoubtedly the condom or guards.

Any other preventives, many of which have been announced with a great flourish, are either useless or even injurious. Injections are particularly to be avoided; they simply serve to carry the gonorrhœal matter which may have been left in the urethra, still farther along in this canal. By observing the rules which we have indicated, infection will be prevented in most cases.

The treatment of gonorrhœa embraces, 1, a regulation of the mode of life, and 2, the therapeutic treatment. A suitable regime is indispensable to a cure. If gonorrhœal patients could be kept at home, in a horizontal position, upon a horse-hair mattrass, chronic gonorrhœa would become a very rare disease.

Let the patient, therefore, remain as quiet as possible; let him avoid all violent exercise, such as dancing, riding on horseback, and likewise every kind of excitement, especially of a sexual nature. The food and beverages he uses, should be without any irritating influence, especially as long as symptoms of inflammation remain visible. He should eat little, and what little he does eat, should be easily digestible. Stool should be had every day. *Cleanliness* is indispensable to a successful cure. The linen and the rags which are tied round the parts, should be changed frequently; the penis and the organs generally should be carefully cleansed with tepid or cold water, and the adhering matter washed off. In washing the parts, all violent friction should be strictly avoided. If the linen should adhere to the orifice of the urethra, it should never be torn off by force, but should first be loosened by soaking it with warm water. If the lips of the orifice should be glued together, and the patient should wish to void urine, care must be had first to free the orifice by moistening it with saliva; otherwise the forcible passage of the stream through the orifice might cause irritation, pain, and even a little hœmorrhage from ruptured capillaries.

In case of inflammatory irritation, tepid local and general baths are to be used, both for purposes of cleanliness, and in order to alleviate the pain and inflammation. But cold baths should be resorted to as soon as the inflammatory symptoms have been subdued, or even from the commencement, if no inflammatory symptoms should at all be present. Water may be drank in quantity, for the purpose of securing a less painful emission of urine, and diminishing the naturally irritating properties of this fluid. Patients who are obliged to be about on account of business, will do well to wear a suspensory. Let us now speak of the medical treatment of this disease.

In gonorrhœa, as well as in any other disease, the homœopathic treatment has decided advantages over the allopathic. However, it is not my intention to mention the large number of remedies which have been recommended by homœopathic physicians, many of them with extravagant praise. I shall simply mention such remedies as have proved efficient in the many cases that I have been called upon to treat. They are the following, together with the symptomatic indications.

Agnus castus is particularly adapted to a yellow purulent discharge from the urethra, after the inflammatory symptoms have subsided for the most part, and in cases of gleet, accompanied by want of erections and deficient sexual desire.

Argentum nitricum is useful when the emission of urine is accompanied by burning, and if a sensation is experienced as though the urethra were closed, and the last portion of the urine remained behind in the urethra; it is also indicated by dragging pains in the urethra, cutting along the urethra as far as the anus, feeling of soreness in the urethra even after micturition, hæmorrhage from the urethra, painful tensive erections, discharge of mucus from the urethra.

Balsamum copaiv. is indicated by smarting pain, burning and itching in the urethra before and after micturition, swelling and inflammation of the orifice of the urethra, painful soreness of the urethra, and purulent discharge from the same.

Cannabis: Smarting pain in the urethra between the acts of micturition, constant urging to urinate, burning and stinging in the urethra, at the corona glandis, and in the outer parts of the prepuce, erections with tensive pains, titillation in the urethra, glueing together of the orifice of the urethra by a moisture which becomes visible on compressing the glans.

Cantharides: Cutting in the urethra during and after micturition; yellowish discharge, which leaves a yellow stain on the linen, and increase of the discharge in secondary gonorrhœa; this agent frequently cuts short the disease when given as soon as the first signs of inflammation become apparent.

Capsicum: Burning at the orifice of the urethra before, during and after micturition, painfulness of the urethra to contact, cutting pain in the urethra between the acts of micturition, pricking as with pins in the forepart of the urethra, thick, purulent, yellow discharge.

Cocculus: Tensive, aching pain in the orifice of the urethra, between the acts of micturition, itching stinging in the forepart of the urethra.

Ferrum: Discharge of mucus from the urethra after a cold.

Mercurius solubilis: Burning pain of the urethra when touching the penis, inflammation of the orifice of the urethra, swelling of the forepart of the urethra with suppuration between the glans and prepuce, redness and heat of the urethra, with painfulness of the same when touching it or when walking, accompanied by a raging pain in the forehead, a feeble stream of the urine, itching and stinging in the forepart of the urethra, throbbing in the same, and a greenish, painless discharge, especially at night, or a slight secretion of moisture from the forepart of the urethra.

Mezereum: Stinging, titillating pain at the urethra and discharge of a little moisture; tearing and drawing through the whole of the urethra, commencing at the perinæum; painful soreness of the urethra when touching it, or partly before, and partly during micturition, and discharge of a watery mucus from the urethra during exercise.

Nux vomica: Pressive pain at the orifice of the urethra between the acts of micturition, accompanied by a feeling of shuddering; sharp pressure, as with a cutting or sticking instrument in the forepart of the urethra, at the bladder, neck of the bladder, perinæum, rectum, anus, as if cutting flatulence were endeavoring to issue from all these parts; accompanied by contractive pains in the forepart of the urethra between the acts of micturition, and discharge of mucus from the urethra depending upon hæmorrhoidal affections.

Petroselinum: Tingling and pressure in the urethra in the region of Cowper's glands, especially early in the morning in bed, abating when standing or sitting; drawing and pressure in the navicular fossa, secretion of a milky fluid from the urethra which can be pressed out; glueing together of the urethra by mucus, discharge of a yellow, glutinous matter from the urethra.

Pulsatilla: Contraction of the urethra and thin stream of the urine, discharge of blood from the urethra, swelling of the testes and inflammation of the eyes caused by suppression of gonorrhœa.

Mercurius corrosivus: Inflammation of the meatus urinarius, itching in the front part of the urethra, smarting pain during micturition, and stitches to and fro in the urethra, with a discharge which is at first thin, afterwards thickly.

Sulphur: Burning in the forepart of the urethra, internally and externally, pains in the urethra at the commencement of gonorrhœa, redness and inflammation of the meatus urinarius, thin stream of the urine, itching in the middle of the urethra, constant desire to urinate, tearing and stinging in the urethra between the acts of micturition, cutting in the urethra before and during stool, and stitches in the forepart of the urethra.

Thuja: Burning in the urethra; burning, piercing stitches near the orifice of the urethra between the acts of micturition, sensation in the urethra as if a drop would run out of it, drawing, cutting pain in the urethra especially when walking, stitches in the urethra from behind forwards between the acts of micturition, jerking pain in the urethra, and a watery, copious discharge.

[*Dose.*—During the acute or inflammatory stage, the tinctures or lower attenuations or lower triturations may be administered, one grain three times a day, or one-third of a drop three times a day, in a spoonful of water or on a little sugar; after the inflammatory symptoms have been subdued, or in the gleetish form of the disease, the middle and higher attenuations may be resorted to, one drop morning and night, and, if a decided improvement is perceived, only one dose every night before retiring. This remark applies to all the remedies and diseases mentioned in this section of the work, as far as SYPHILITIC DISEASES PROPER.]

Balannorrhœa, balanitis, balanoposthitis.

By balanorrhœa we understand an inflammation and a purulent secretion on the surface of the glans and on the inner side of the prepuce, a condition which may arise from gonorrhœal infection as well as from the action of non-contagious irritating causes.

This secretion emanates from the follicular glands situated behind the corona glandis and which, even in health, secrete a cheesy, strong-smelling substance.

The disease generally runs the following course: at first the patients experience a slight smarting or burning on the surface of the glans or in the prepuce. The parts, especially the glans, are hot, of a rose color or a bright carmine redness, somewhat swollen, sensitive to pressure and especially to the rubbing of the clothes when walking. The follicular secretion is very much increased; it soon becomes purulent, thick, greenish-yellow. The pus is discharged on each side of the frænulum in large tenacious drops. The margin of the prepuce is swollen, bright-red, somewhat distended; both it and the folds of the prepuce are constantly filled with pus which sometimes dries up, forming small crusts of a dirty yellow color, and causing the prepuce to adhere to the linen. The inner surface of the prepuce has an intensely bright-red color. Upon this inner surface as well as upon the glans, we soon notice erosions of the mucous membrane having a red or grayish-red color, and readily becoming gangrenous and inducing violent incidental affections, such as phymosis, paraphymosis, which will be described bye and bye. The flat little ulcers are not syphilitic, and are caused by the acridity of the secreted matter. In most cases they remain unchanged for a week or a fortnight, after which the cure is rapidly effected.

A benign balannorrhœa frequently occurs in children, but principally in individuals with a long prepuce which is not entirely drawn behind the glans during coït, on which account the pus which has penetrated between it and the glans is enabled to remain without being disturbed. However, balannorrhœa may likewise occur when the prepuce is short or even entirely wanting. Circumcised persons are free from it almost entirely. This secretion is not contagious.

The venereal or contagious balannorrhœa is contracted during coït. It is of rare occurrence, notwithstanding that the surface of the glans is sooner exposed to the contagious pus than the urethra.

This circumstance may be owing to the peculiar nature of the epithelium of the glans, and to the fact that the pus adheres to it but a short time, and is then wiped off again. It generally shows itself sooner than gonorrhœa, sometimes one or two hours, but in most cases from three to six days after an impure coït.

In regard to preventive means, the same rules should be followed that we have laid down in treating of gonorrhœa; cleanliness, washing the parts with soap and water after intercourse, and all the other precautionary rules are indispensable.

In regard to regime and diet, the same rules have to be followed that have been mentioned for gonorrhœa.

Of the remedies used the following were found the most efficient: *Acidum Nitricum*, *Cannabis*, *Capsicum*, *China*, *Cinnabaris*, *Mercurius solubilis*, *Mezereum*, *Nux vomica*, *Pulsatilla*, *Sabina*, *Stannum*, *Sulphur*, and *Thuja*. The following are the symptomatic indications:

Acidum Nitricum: Balannorrhœa with small vesicles in the orifice of the uretha, on the inner surface, and at the margin of the prepuce; they soon break, suppurate, and form chancrous ulcers; or with brown, painful, lentil-sized spots on the glans, excavated ulcers on the glans, with elevated, lead-colored, sensitive margins; flat, clean little ulcers at the corona glandis, secreting a strong-smelling matter; flesh-colored excrescences at the corona glandis, secreting a fetid humor and bleeding when touched; itching of the prepuce, and humid spots on its inner surface, and sharp stinging pains in the same.

Cannabis: The glans is covered with small bright-red spots, which are lighter than the glans itself when the glans is as red as the prepuce; redness and dampness behind the corona glandis; itching under the prepuce, and at the frænulum; swelling of the glans and penis, like a sort of painless erection; dampness round the corona glandis; constant burning of the prepuce and glans.

Capsicum: Constant pressure and prickling in the glans; fine itching, stinging of the glans as if bit by mosquitoes.

China: Burning in the glans, and creeping and pressure in the urethra and anus; itching of the glans, especially in the evening in bed; twitching pain between the glans and prepuce during a walk; tearing pain in the left side of the prepuce, and in the left testicle; fine pricking at the frænulum as with pins.

Cinnabaris: Burning, stinging, itching of the corona glandis; itching pain in the fossa behind the glans, with exudation of pus of a nauseous sweetish smell; tearing stitches in the glans; small red spots on the glans; or red shining little dots or readily-bleeding warts on the prepuce.

Mercurius solubilis: Burning around the glans, followed by the breaking out of vesicles on the inner surface of the prepuce, which soon break and give rise to small ulcers, with itching stinging in the glans after pressure; tearing stitching pain in the fore-part of the glans, extending through the whole penis as far as behind the anus, and sometimes even as far as the groins; vesicles on the fore-part of the glans, on the upper surface, and at the sides, penetrating and spreading, and discharging an acrid humor; suppuration between the glans and prepuce, with swelling of the fore-part of the urethra, which looks red and feels hot, and is very painful when touched or during exercise; ulcers on the glans and prepuce, with a cheesy, lardaceous bottom, and a hard margin; swelling of the glans and prepuce; tingling at the frænulum and scrotum; fine red eruption on the outer, and cracks and rhagades on the inner surface of the swollen prepuce.

Mezereum: Itching, tearing and twitching tearing in the glans; fine prickling stitches in the penis and at the tip of the glans; tearing drawing at the corona glandis, with secretion of a quantity of yellowish smegma in that region, and inflammatory redness of the prepuce which exhibits excoriations, accompanied by a feeling of soreness in the glans and prepuce.

Nux vomica: Smarting and burning itching of the glans, copious secretion of smegma behind the corona glandis; smarting itching of the inner side of the prepuce, especially towards evening.

Pulsatilla: Smarting and corrosive itching of the glans under the prepuce; agreeable titillation of the glans, accompanied by a discharge of a colorless mucus; constrictive pain behind the glans; itching, smarting pain of the inner and upper portion of the prepuce; finely stinging itching in the prepuce when sitting or lying.

Sabina: Burning soreness of the glans when touching it; dark redness of the glans; painfulness of the prepuce, and inability to press it back behind the glans; occasional turns of pain at the frænulum.

Stannum: Burning pain in the glans, followed by urging to urinate; burning prickings in the glans.

Sulphur: Swelling, redness and coldness of the prepuce and glans, accompanied by stitches in the penis.

Thuja: Burning itching, with a feeling of soreness and stitches in the glans; titillating sensation between the prepuce and glans; violent stitches in the glans near the urethra, which are always accompanied by an urging to urinate, the urine passing off in drops, the stitches are at times very violent, and at other times they disappear altogether; red spots and erosions on the corona glandis, which become moist and suppurate; flat, unclean, red ulcers, with burning pain at the corona glandis; dampness of the glans, with acutely-painful stitches in the interior of the prepuce, and smooth, red excrescences in the region where the prepuce adheres to the body of the penis.

Affections which accompany Gonorrhœa and Blennorrhœa.

These accessory affections are in direct relation with the gonorrhœal discharge. They are either caused by it, or supervene by chance. We will mention these accessory affections seriatim, give a brief description of their phenomena, and indicate the remedies by which they are removed.

I. Erections.

These are present in almost every case of gonorrhœa, and frequently cause the most violent pains. They always aggravate the inflammatory condition. They are more painful during a first attack of gonorrhœa than in those who had been several times attacked with this disease.

The patient should not only observe the rules which have been laid down for the cure of gonorrhœa, but he should guard against every mental or bodily excitement, and more particularly against lascivious fancies. He should never feel of his parts; eat very little supper or none at all; sleep on a horse-hair mattrass; not lie on his back; void the urine frequently, even at night, in order to avoid every possible pressure and irritation of the seminal vesicles.

The principal remedies will be found to be *Capsicum* and *Cantharides*, or one of the remedies mentioned for gonorrhœa, to be selected in accordance with the symptoms.

II. Satyriasis and Priapism.

Satyriasis (or a frantic desire for coït in the male) and priapism, (or a painful erection of the penis,) are conditions of the parts where the erections never cease, and are accompanied by an excessive degree of sexual excitement. For such conditions we recommend cold hip-baths, cold water bandages round the parts, and the internal use of *Agaricus, Petroselinum, Cantharides, Acidum phosphoricum, Opium and Hyoscyamus.*

III. Chordee.

On account of the violent inflammation, the longitudinal muscles of the urethra and the erector muscles are not put upon the stretch simultaneously. The patients complain of a sensation as though the penis were curved by force. This curvature or twisting actually takes place; sometimes the penis is bent downwards, sometimes upwards, and at other times laterally. These phenomena of an intensely-developed inflammation may extend even to the corpus spongiosum. If this inflammation is not subdued in season, it may terminate in some chronic disorganisation, thickening, indurations and adhesions. If adhesions have taken place, a cure can no longer be expected. The chordee then remains a permanent condition of the parts, coït is more or less painful, and sometimes even impossible.

Among the lower classes, the custom still prevails here and there to beat the penis, in order to remove the chordee; they place the concave side upon a table, and strike the convex portion with their fist; it need scarcely be told, that this violent proceeding sometimes results in distressing consequences.

Suitable means for the cure of this affection are cold baths and hip-baths, vapor-baths, the use of the north-pole of the magnet, the internal use of *Capsicum, Cantharides, Chamomilla* and *Pulsatilla.*

IV. Hæmorrhage from the Urethra.

In very violent inflammations, a discharge of blood may be useful, for it has been observed, that the inflammatory symptoms abated afterwards, and that even the chordee ceased. Excessive hæmorrhage is undoubtedly hurtful, and should be arrested. The patient should be kept in a horizontal posture, the penis should be compressed; cold water or ice should be applied to the penis, and internally the following remedies should be resorted to: *Acidum nitricum*, *Argentum nitricum*, *Cantharides*. [I have found *Aconite* useful in many cases, Ed.]

V. Inflammation of Cowper's Glands.

This is indicated by a pain and swelling of the perinæum. It should be subdued as soon as possible, for it is apt to terminate in inflammation. If the suppuration has already set in, it must be promoted, and means afforded for the pus to escape, lest an urinary fistula should develope itself.

As soon as the first signs of inflammation make their appearance, we should administer *Mercurius solubilis*, *Sulphur* or *Thuja*.

VI. Prostatitis, Inflammation of the Prostate Gland.

This inflammation commences with a sensation of pressure and heat in the perinæum, towards the neck of the bladder and rectum. The patients complain of a continual and painful urging to pass urine and stool; likewise of a sensation as if some foreign body had lodged in the rectum. The pain increases with every attempt to satisfy the urging, which is either fruitless or results in a very scanty discharge. This inflammation very frequently runs a chronic course.

In acute cases the following remedies are indicated: *Aconite*, *Belladonna*, *Bryonia*, *Cannabis*, *Mercurius solubilis*, *Phosphorus*, *Thuja*; they have to be selected in accordance with the symptoms.

VII. Dysuria.

This is invariably present in every case of gonorrhœa, where the posterior portions of the urethra are affected. We give, according to the symptoms, *Cantharides*, *Copaiva*, *Mercurius solubilis*, *Thuja*.

If the urinary tenesmus should continue and a dangerous

result should have to be apprehended, the catheter may have to be introduced. The operation should be performed with great caution, lest a false passage should be made.

Affections which may occur without Gonorrhœa.

There is a class of affections which sometimes accompany the gonorrhœal discharge, but may likewise occur in connection with, or without any other morbid conditions. These are

I. Pruritus Glandis, itching of the Glans.

Sometimes the patients complain of an intolerable itching of the glans which induces such a violent scratching that the itching parts and those which surround them, are frequently rendered sore by the scratching. This itching consists in an increased irritability of the parts, is sometimes extremely obstinate, and is apt to recur. It not only occurs during and after the existence of gonorrhœa, but also in cases where neither gonorrhœa nor ulcers had existed, and where the parts had indeed never been affected by any disease.

I have employed with the greatest success, *Antimonium crudum*, *Causticum*, *Arsenic*, *Calcarea sulph.*

The itching may likewise be experienced by females who have the whites or even by such as are perfectly healthy, or even by girls of the most unexceptionable conduct during or after the menses. The same remedies which have been mentioned previously, will help in the case of females.

II. Eczema, Herpes Præputialis.

This troublesome vesicular eruption may affect both sexes either with or without a syphilitic taint. In the male these vesicles are located on the prepuce and glans, in the female on the labia majora and minora. The inexperienced physician might easily mistake them for incipient chancre. It is therefore of the greatest importance to be well acquainted with them. Sometimes the prepuce looks red in one or more places, the redness extending over a larger or smaller space. Generally the patients are not aware of the disease until their attention is directed to it by the itching of the red and swollen parts. The fully developed vesicles are of the size of a pin's head, never larger.

Generally several of these vesicles are clustered together, sometimes they run into each other. By using one or the other of the following remedies, which have to be selected with reference to the totality of the perceptible symptoms, these vesicles generally dry up and disappear after the lapse of from four to five days, after which the itching ceases: *Acidum phosphoricum*, *Petroleum*, *Thuja*. If these vesicles break out previous to the monthly period, we may add: *Veratrum*, at other times *Mercurius sol.*

III. Œdema præputii, Swelling of the Prepuce.

Gonorrhœa is sometimes accompanied by a swelling of the prepuce caused by infiltration and exudation of a serous fluid. If this swelling is opened, a clear, and sometimes a bloody serum is discharged, frequently in large quantity. The prepuce looks dark-red, hot, inflamed, and the swelling is sometimes so considerable that it looks like a bladder distended by air or water. In the former case, *Cannabis* and *Sulpur* are the remedies, in the latter *Merc. sol.*

IV. Phymosis.

This affection is closely related to the last-named condition, and is frequently caused by it. It is a contraction or constriction of the prepuce in front of the glans, so that it is either impossible or extremely difficult to pull the prepuce over the glans. It arises from an inflammation of the subcutaneous cellular tissue of the prepuce, in which a quantity of serum is deposited. The external layer of the prepuce has the usual color, is smooth, shining; the internal mucous membrane is of a rose color, transparent, the prepuce is considerably swollen, and the glans is likewise enlarged. These circumstances sufficiently account for the impossibility of denuding the glans.

Phymosis never takes place without balannorrhœa; out of

every ten cases of balannorrhœa, one is generally accompanied by phymosis. Generally only such men are affected by this disease as are troubled with a long and narrow prepuce even during health. Among circumcised persons this disease is impossible.

Sometimes the swelling and inflammation of the prepuce increase so rapidly that gangrene may set in. The prepuce forms a large, long, dark brown-red bulbous swelling at the extremity of the penis; its borders are enlarged like thick lips, cracked and so narrow that only a small portion of the secreted pus, which is generally thin, and sometimes thick, and of a green-yellow color, can flow out; the remainder of the pus collects behind the corona glandis, where it forms an indistinctly fluctuating swelling.

The pain is very acute. In some cases the remaining portion of the integuments of the penis, as far as the root, and even the skin of the scrotum and of the inguinal region, are involved in the inflammation.

Among the homœopathic remedies with which this affection should be treated, we distinguish: *Merc. sol.*, *Rhus t. Thuja*, *Cannabis*, *Cinnabaris*, *Sulphur* and *Viola tri-color*. If these remedies should not effect a cure, it may be necessary to make slight incisions into the prepuce, for the purpose of allowing the fluid to escape; in extremely difficult cases, when gangrene threatens, it may be necessary to remove the long and unyielding prepuce with the knife.

V. Paraphymosis.

In this affection the constriction of the prepuce takes place behind the glans. The prepuce is generally inverted, and the outer skin is more or less covered by the inner membrane. If the constriction is not speedily removed, the inflammation soon reaches a dangerous height, and invades the whole penis.

We treat this disease with *Cannabis*, *Sabina*, *Mercurius sol.*, and, in dangerous cases, we may have to resort to the operation.

Sequelæ of Gonorrhœa.

Beside the accessory or secondary affections of gonorrhœa, of which we have treated in the preceding chapters, we have a series of affections which are the sequelæ of gonorrhœa, to which they owe, more or less, their origin.

The sequelæ of gonorrhœa may be divided into two classes, those which arise from a metastasis of gonorrhœal inflammation to other organs, and secondly, those which are characterised by disorganizations or functional derangements of the organs that are sympathetically affected during the course of gonorrhœa.

Affections caused by a Metastasis of the Gonorrhœal Inflammation of other Organs.

I. Glandular swellings in the Groin, Gonorrhœal Buboes.

These swellings occur in many cases of gonorrhœa. In most cases of violent gonorrhœa the inguinal glands are more or less sensitive, even if not much swollen or inflamed. At first they constitute moveable little tumors of the size of beans, rather hard, painful when walking. At this stage it is still possible to scatter them by treatment. By neglect they become inflamed, grow larger, and then form the buboes properly speaking.

These buboes may either be the result of con-sensual or sympathetic irritation, or they may be an indication of genuine syphilis. These two forms of bubo require to be distinguished with great care. We will here describe the former variety; the second form will be treated of in the chapters on primary syphilis.

In the case of a gonorrhœal bubo, the cellular tissue which surrounds the gland, first begins to swell. Gradually this swelling increases, suppuration sets in, the skin becomes red, the patients experience a drawing and tension in the inguinal region, pressure on the tumor causes pain, walking becomes more troublesome; finally the swelling grows softer, the skin over the swelling breaks, and a thick yellow pus, or a thin yellowish fluid is discharged, with disks of pus floating in it.

These glandular swellings supervene in the first fortnight, while the gonorrhœal inflammation is still confined to the region of the navicular fossa. They are caused by the pus being absorbed by the lymphatics of the penis, which carry it to the glands where it causes an inflammation. The development of buboes is hastened by much bodily exercise or fatiguing efforts during the inflammatory stage of gonorrhœa.

As regards the treatment of buboes, during the early stage of inflammation and swelling, the patient should remain as quiet as possible, and take one of the following remedies: *Aconite*, *Belladonna*, *Carbo anim.*, *Lycopod.*, *Merc. sol.*, *Phosph.*, *Rhus t.*, *Thuja*.

[*Aconite*, more particularly, if the inflammation is very acute, and accompanied by fever;

Belladonna, after the fever begins to decline, and a subacute stage of the inflammation has developed itself;

Mercurius sol., if the swelling is neither red nor very sore, and has developed itself very slowly;

Rhus tox., when the tumor is as hard as stone, and almost insensible;

Lycopod. and *Thuja*, if the tumor has become chronic after one or more of the other remedies had been used.]

If the increased redness and the presence of fluctuation should lead us to infer that pus has been formed, the suppurative process should be hastened by the application of warm poultices; internally one of the following remedies which are physiologically related to the morbid process, may be given: *Belladonna*, *Hepar sulph.*, *Merc. sol.*, *Silicea*. If the inflammation and the pain should be very violent, and the tumor should not break voluntarily, the patient will derive great relief from the tumor being lanced.

II. Cystitis, Inflammation of the Bladder.

This disease is not very frequent. It arises from the mucous membrane of the neck of the bladder, or even the bladder, being invaded by the gonorrhœal inflammation. It is generally accompanied with inflammation of the prostate gland. The patients complain of distressing pains in the region of the bladder, causing a good deal of oppressive anxiety and spreading to the adjoining parts, the perinæum, anus, testicles, loins. The pains and the anguish are still increased by the violent urinary tenesmus, in consequence of which the urine can only be discharged in drops. These phenomena are of course accompanied by violent fever, the patients spend sleepless and distressing nights, and lose strength and flesh. The urine is turbid, and deposits a bloody and purulent sediment.

A very strict diet is here rendered necessary by the intensity of the inflammation. The following remedies may be exhibited: *Aconite*, *Acidum phosphor.*, *Bryonia*, *Staphys.*, *Tart. emet.*, and *Veratr.*

[The principal remedies are undoubtedly *Aconite* and *Cantharides*, which may be used alternately, in tincture form, two or three drops of the *Aconite*, and one drop of *Cantharides*, in separate tumblerfuls of water, a tablespoonful of each solution every half hour alternately, until the dangerous and distressing symptoms have abated, after which the medicines may be continued at longer intervals, every hour or two hours. If, after the subsidence of all the acute symptoms, some strangury should still remain,

Nux vomica or *Pulsatilla* may be resorted to, and then again Aconite or Cantharides, or both in alternation, until the cure is completed.]

III. Epididymitis Blennorrhagica, Acute Inflammation of the Epididymis.

This disease is one of the most frequently-occurring complications of gonorrhœa, and, on account of the cause whence it springs, one of the most important. It is either caused by the spread of the gonorrhœal inflammation along the ejaculatory canal and the vas deferens, so that the spermatic cord is simultaneously invaded by the inflammatory process, or by sympathy, in which case these last-mentioned organs are not affected. Many contend that such an inflammation may be caused by a sudden suppression of the gonorrhœal discharge. This opinion is contradicted by other authorities of the highest standing. Ricord especially asserts that the best preventive of inflammation of the testes is a speedy removal of the gonorrhœal discharge; and that this inflammation occurs most frequently in cases where the gonorrhœa had not been treated at all. Orchitis frequently occurs simultaneously with gonorrhœa, but most frequently in the last stage of the disease.

Orchitis is more readily superinduced when the following conditions occur: excessive afflux of venous blood to the testes, relaxation of the scrotum, large size of the testes, frequent voluntary or involuntary emissions of semen, sexual excitement, or else unnatural abstemiousness, efforts and irritations of the neighboring parts by standing, walking, riding, vesical calculi, constipation, colds, mechanical injuries such as blows, contusions, etc. Improper medical treatment, such as irritating injections, may likewise occasion this disease.

It generally runs the following course: after the gonorrhœa has continued for a while, the patient experiences a sensation of pressure and heaviness either immediately in the testes, or first in the region of the kidneys, groins, perinæum. The pain increases, particularly if the testicle is left to its weight, or by standing; and, if it reaches a high degree, it extends to the thigh, abdomen and small of the back. Colicky pains set in, accompanied by urinary difficulties; even the peritoneum may be invaded. Sometimes the spermatic cord swells to such a degree that it becomes constricted, and phenomena resembling those of incarcerated hernia, develope themselves. If the disease is violent, there is always some fever. The sensitiveness of the affective parts is sometimes so great that the least contact of the parts causes the patients to faint away.

The disease runs a very rapid course, and an appropriate treatment removes it in a few days.

The treatment is both prophylactic and curative. The prophylactic treatment prescribes a strict avoidance of all sexual excitement from the moment that the gonorrhœa first shows itself, and of every exposure or influence that might give rise to orchitis. The patient should wear a suitable suspensory until one or two weeks after the gonorrhœa has ceased.

The internal treatment is to be conducted with one or more of the following remedies :

Aconite: Contusive pain in the testicle, with fever.

Acidum nitricum: Swelling and inflammation of the testes, whence the pain travels to the abdomen through the spermatic cords; the testicle is painful to contact, with tearing in the spermatic cord.

Acidum phosphoricum: Aching pain in both testes, worse when waking or when touching the parts; burning tearing in the left testicle, and burning in the prostate gland, with frequent erections.

Ammonium carbon.: Strangling pain in the testes and spermatic cords, with sensitiveness of the testes to contact and involuntary erections; seminal emissions preceded by a drawing and strangling sensation in the testes.

Argentum nitricum: Contusive pain, with enlargement and hardness of the right testicle.

Arsenicum: Crampy cutting colic darting through the abdominal ring and the perinæum, considerable swelling of the testicles, phenomena resembling those of incarcerated hernia.

Aurum: Swelling of the lower part of the right testicle, with an aching pain when touching or rubbing the part; aching tensive pain in the right testicle, as if contused.

Baryt acet.: Frequently recurring and disappearing swelling of the testicles.

Belladonna: Tearing in the left spermatic cord, especially in the evening, in bed, previous to falling asleep; drawing in the spermatic cord during the acts of micturition; long stitches in the testicle which is drawn up.

Bismuth: Aching pain in the right testicle, worse when touching the part.

Cannabis: Tensive pain in the spermatic cord and contraction of the scrotum, or contractive sensation in the scrotum when standing; sensation of pressure in the testicles, or a pulling sensation.

Cantharides: Drawing pain in the spermatic cord during micturition, with swelling of the scrotum.

Capsicum: Drawing pain in the spermatic cord, and a crampy pain in the testicle during and some time after micturition.

Causticum: Aching pain in the testicles, stitches in the right testicle.

China: Painful swelling of the spermatic cord and testicle, especially of the epididymis; tearing pain in the left testicle and in the left side of the prepuce, a crampy-contractive pain in the testicles and urethra, especially in the evening.

Clematis: Swelling of both testes; ascending pain in the testicle and spermatic cord.

Cocculus: Stitching pain in one or the other testicle; violent pains in both testicles as if bruised, especially during contact; drawing pain in the testicles.

Colocynthis: Continual violent drawing in the left testicle, painful twitching of the testes, they are drawing up.

Ignatia: Pressure in the testicles; severe strangling sensation in the testicles, in the evening after lying down in bed.

Iodium: Swelling and induration of the testes and prostate gland.

Ipecacuanha: Twisting, drawing pain in the testicle.

Marum verum: Descension of the right spermatic cord towards the abdominal ring, with a sensation as if the spermatic cord were pressed; crampy sensation deep in the abdomen, which extends to the testicles as if they had been violently pressed upon; the integuments of the left testicle feel sore when touched, as if a pain had invaded them, starting from the root of the penis.

North-pole of the magnet: Cutting and sharp drawing in the testes; sharp stitches in the left testicle; strangling pain in the right testicle; sharp drawing and cutting in the testicles.

South-pole of the magnet: Tearing in the spermatic cord; pain in the spermatic cord, early in the morning, while the testicle is hanging down relaxed, as if the cord were pulled upon; the testicle is painful when touched; slow, fine, painful drawing in the spermatic cord; swelling of the testicles, and a tearing, strangling jerk in the same; at night the testes are spasmodically drawn up.

Manganum aceticum: Aching, drawing pain in the spermatic cord, as if drawn up, and in the testicles, with a feeling of weakness in the parts.

Magnes.: Swelling of the epididymis, and simple pain in the same when touching it, or during motion.

Mercurius solub.: Paroxysmal drawing in the spermatic cord; sensitiveness of the swollen testicle, which, however, is not painful; feeling of coldness in the testes; itching in the right testicle; crampy, tearing pain, commencing between the testes, afterwards penetrating into the penis and causing a good deal of itching; drawing pain in the testicles and in the groin; drawing with pressure, the drawing being the most distressing.

Mezereum: Painless swelling of the left testicle, which had been swollen in former times.

Nux vomica: Heat in the testes; stitches in the same; contractive pain in the testicles.

Oleum anim.: Alternate swelling of one or the other testicles, with pain when touched.

Pulsatilla: Swelling of the right spermatic cord and testicles, with a tensive pain. Drawing pains, and drawing tensive pains pass out of the abdomen through the spermatic cord into the testicles which are relaxed. The right testicle is drawn up and swollen, with a tensive pain, whereas the left testicle is hanging down relaxed. The testes and spermatic cords are painful and swollen, with discharge of prostatic fluid; tearing pain in the testes; the testicles hang down very loosely, with tensive, drawing pains passing out the abdomen into the testicles through the spermatic cord.

Rhododendron: Distressing pain in the testicles, especially in the epididymis, when touching the parts; the testicles are drawn up and swollen; contusive pain of the testes.

Spigelia: Stitching pain in one testicle; itching stinging in the left testicle; itching stitch in the right testicle and in the penis from behind forward; burning stitch in the right testicle and in the penis.

Spongia marina: Painfulness and swelling of the spermatic cord; long dull stitches proceeding from the spermatic cord and striking into the testes; painful aching swelling of the testes and spermatic cords; the testicle is painful when touched; crampy, strangulating, contusive pain in the right testicle.

Staphysagria: Violent, drawing-burning stitches from the right spermatic cord to the right testicle through the abdominal ring, when sitting, walking or standing, most violent when stooping; aching pain in the left testicle, aggravated by walking and by contact or friction; drawing and tearing in the right testicle, with pressure, as if it were forcibly compressed.

Sulphur: Pressure and tension in the spermatic cords and testicles; slow tingling in the testicles, all day; sometimes a slight buzzing is experienced in the thighs, whence it passes to the testes, after which it recommences as before, more violently; vibratory sensation in the testicles and other organs.

Thuja: Burning stitches with pressure from below upwards, through the scrotum and spermatic cord; drawing and stitching in the spermatic cords and in the testicles; aching pain in the testicles, as if contused, when walking or sitting.

Zincum: Frequent drawing in the testes, following the course of the spermatic cord. Painfulness and swelling of the testes. Drawing pricking pain in the testes, worse when sitting or stooping.

IV. Ophthalmia Gonorrhœica.

This affection arises from the metastasis of the gonorrhœal discharge to the eye, the discharge remaining either unaltered, or becoming less, or entirely suppressed. This disease occurs more frequently among men than women, and generally affects one eye only. The conjunctiva is not much affected, the disease generally develops itself slowly. In blepharophthalmitis gonorrhœica the redness and swelling of the conjunctiva are generally very moderate; the secretion is of the same quality as in the common blennorrhœa of the eyes, but less in quantity, and the pain is less likewise.

In the very acute and rapidly-developed form of ophthalmia gonorrhœica, we distinctly observe three stages. The first stage sets in with a violent, burning itching especially at the margins of the lids and in the canthi, accompanied by a profuse flow of acrid tears, and considerable photophobia; the conjunctiva is uniformly reddened, and the lids, especially the upper ones, swell considerably. In the region where the conjunctiva passes from the lids to the eyeball, a good deal of vascular engorgement takes place. Towards the end of this stage, which generally is of short duration, the tears become more turbid. These phenomena are accompanied by fever, dulness of the head, coated tongue and violent thirst.

In a few days the second stage commences with considerable swelling of the conjunctiva; at first a whitish yellow mucus, to which the tears with which it is mixed, impart a watery consistence, is secreted; it speedily increases in quantity and thickness, assumes a greenish tint after a while, and, in flowing down the cheeks, either inflames or corrodes them. The upper lid sometimes swells to the size of a hen's egg, the lower lid is less swollen. The pains become extremly acute, and from the eye and its surrounding parts spread over the whole head. The conjunctiva which looks red as far as the cornea, forms a pad-shaped elevation around the cornea, covering its margins, and penetrating even as a dark-red mass between the lids which become everted in consequence, especially the lower. There is a profuse secretion of mucus from the conjunctiva, the inflammation speedily invades the cornea whose interstices become distended even in a few hours, and which assumes an uniformly grayish or yellowish appearance.

The fever, in the second stage, is of course worse; the raging pain causes sleeplessness, and even delirium.

If this stage is not arrested by artificial means, the third stage sets in, and with it a complete disorganization of the cornea by suppuration. In consequence of this destruction the eye frequently breaks and the whole of the contents of the interior eye are discharged; or else ulcerations of the cornea take place here and there.

When the third stage has set in, the pains in and around the eye decrease, the mucus becomes less, more watery, yellowish-white, less corrosive; the swelling of the eyelids and of the conjunctiva decreases, the whites begin to reappear, and the phlyctænæ of the cornea dry up. The fever ceases entirely, but all sorts of disorganizations remain, such as: prolapsus of the iris, adhesions of the iris and cornea, staphyloma, leucoma, disturbances of the visual power, dimness of the lenticular capsule, adhesions of the capsule to the margin of the pupil.

The course of this disease varies according to the constitution of the patient. In young and robust persons it is rapid, in old and debilitated individuals it runs a slow course.

The causes of ophthalmic gonorrhœa are—1, *direct poisoning of the eye with gonorrhœal matter*; 2, *metastasis of the gonorrhœal discharge to the eye after complete suppression or considerable decrease of the discharge*; and 3, *spreading of the inflammation to the conjunctiva as to a homogeneous tissue.*

The opinions of authors respecting this disease vary a good deal. St. Yves and Plenk consider metastasis as the only cause of the disease. Richter, Beer, Walther, Dupuytren,

Schœn, Himly, attribute only the more acute form of this disease to metastasis; Howard, Foot, Spangenberg, Ritter, Benedict, Lawrence and others, on the contrary, derive it from some local infection; Ricord likewise denies ever having seen it take place after suppression of the original discharge.

It is conceded that the more acute forms of gonorrhœic ophthalmia are caused by the gonorrhœic poison getting into the eye; this accounts for the fact that men are more frequently attacked by the disease than women, and that only one eye, principally the right one, is generally affected; for the patients are in the habit of touching the diseased parts with the right hand, and afterwards rubbing with it the right eye for the purpose of stopping the itching which they may happen to experience.

Suppression of gonorrhœa is undoubtedly the least frequent cause of ophthalmia gonorrhœica.

The prognosis in this disease is generally very unfavorable. The visual power can only be preserved by a suitable treatment being instituted from the commencement. If the inflammation should be far advanced, the cornea considerably affected, interstitially distended, covered with phlyctænæ, considerable disturbances of the visual power can scarcely be prevented. It is therefore advisable, according to Ricord, to look upon every case of ophthalmia which takes place simultaneously with gonorrhœa as a malignant form of inflammation, and to institute a treatment accordingly.

As regards treatment, the use of specific remedies should be accompanied by the observance of the strictest cleanliness.

Even in the lesser forms of the disease, the affected eye should be used as little as possible, and should be protected by a screen against the light.

In the commencement of the disease *Aconite* is an excellent remedy; in the lighter forms it alone frequently effects a cure.

In violent inflammation, with burning pains, copious discharge of mucus, one or more from among the following remedies should be used: *Arg. nit.*, *Belladonna*, *Calomel*,

Cannabis, *Carbo veget.* *Euphrasia*, *Graphites*, *Hepar sulph.*, *Lycopod.*, *Merc. sol.*, *Nitric acid*, *Mercurius corrosivus*, *Sulphur*, *Tart. emet.*, *Thuja*, *Verat. alb.*

In inveterate cases *Tussilago petasites* has been found useful. In cases where the iris had become affected, which is frequently the case when matter gets into the eye, *China*, *Colchicum*, *Euphorbium*, *Sulphur* and *Terebinth.*, will be found efficacious remedies.

[The principal remedies are undoubtedly *Aconite*, *Acidum nitricum* and the mercurial preparations, especially *Mercurius præcipitatus ruber*, *corrosivus*, *dulcis* and *acetatus*.

Aconite, when the inflammation is very acute, and the pains in the eye and in the region of the eyebrows agonizing, cutting, throbbing, burning, with excessive sensitiveness to the light; after the acute pains have been subdued by Aconite, and this agent does not seem any longer to act in the case, we may resort to

Belladonna, for aching, sore pains, with sensitiveness to the light, dilated pupils, frontal headache; or

Euphrasia, when the inflammation is accompanied by a profuse secretion of tears;

Acidum nitricum, when the anterior chamber seems filled with a dirty-looking pus, as if the eye would become disorganized.

The mercurial preparations may be used in the following order: corrosivus, dulcis, ruber, and lastly, acetatus, for symptoms of disorganization, opacity or ulceration of the cornea, opacity of the lens, distortion of the pupil. If symptoms of iritis develope themselves during the acute attack, *Aconite* in alternation with *Mercurius corrosivus* are invaluable agents; of the Aconite, mixing three or four drops of the saturated tincture of the root in a tumblerful of water, and giving the corrosive mercury in grain doses of the third trituration.]

V. Gonorrhœa of the Buccal and Nasal Cavities.

It is supposed that the gonorrhœal matter may be carried to the nasal cavity by means of the pocket-handkerchief, and that in consequence inflammation of and discharge from the nostrils may take place. It appears, however, that this form of the disease occurs very seldom. It has only been observed by few authors. At first the symptoms are like those of a common catarrh; afterwards the mucous membrane swells, and the discharge becomes purulent and profuse.

Actual gonorrhœa has likewise been noticed from the buccal cavity. Such cases are related by Petrosi, of Kiel, and Sigmund, of Vienna; both men and women have had their mouths infected with the gonorrhœal disease by bringing these parts in contact with the contagious matter.—Petrosi relates as follows: A young man was attacked with gonorrhœa of the urethra, and, in consequence of applying his mouth to the diseased pudendum, the buccal cavity likewise became diseased. Already on the following day he experienced a pain about the lips and gums. On the fourth day the mucous membrane of the lips and buccal cavity became intensely red; the motions of the mouth became painful; the gums were interstitially distended, receding from the teeth, readily bleeding, and the secretions from the buccal cavity were more copious. Afterwards a copious, purulent, tenacious and ropy secretion, with aphthous exudations under the tongue, and painful deglutition set in. Professor Sigmund, indeed, admits that, in most cases, the gonorrhœal disease of the mouth arises from the poisonous matter of the same person being brought in contact with the lips; however, he mentions cases where the disease was caused by introducing the diseased penis into the mouth of another person, or by licking the affected pudendum with the tongue. Sigmund not believing it possible that human degeneracy could reach this low level, an experienced prostitute afforded him an opportunity of being an unseen witness of such an act perpetrated by an old frequenter of haunts of vice.

The strictest cleanliness is likewise required for a successful treatment of nasal and buccal gonorrhœa. The internal treatment of the gonorrhœal inflammation of the mucous membrane of the nose and mouth requires the use of *Aurum*, *Calcarea*, *Hepar sulph.*, *Pulsatilla*, *Phosphorus*, *Mercurius corrosivus*, *Sulphur* and *Thuja.*

[*Aurum*, when the discharge from the nose is very offensive and the internal parts of the nose feel very sore. If this should not help, resort to

Hepar sulphuris, especially if the discharge is of an acrid and excoriating nature; if thin and ichorous, burning,

Arsenic may be given; or, if attended with swelling, inflammation, soreness of the nostrils,

Mercurius corrosivus and *Sulphur* in alternation.]

VI. Gonorrhœa of the Rectum.

This form of gonorrhœa may be caused by an unnatural gratification of the sexual instinct, or in the case of females, by the gonorrhœal matter flowing from the vagina downwards along the perinæum into the anal fissure; in any case, the disease is caused by direct contact of the poison. In the case of females, where it is caused by self-infection, the skin around the anus is generally inflamed, excoriated, secreting a turbid, purulent fluid. In large cities it is rather frequent, particularly among prostitutes and men given to Sodomitic habits.

Cleanliness and one or more of the following remedies will cure the disease: *Aconite*, *Argentum*, *Aurum*, *Belladonna*, *Calcarea*, *Ignatia*, *Merc. sol.*, *Natr. mur.*, *Nux vom.*, *Phosphorus*, *Sepia* and *Sulphur.*

[*Aconite*, for burning, shooting pains, with soreness and inflammation.

Mercurius, for stitching pains, with purulent discharge.

Nux vomica and *Sulphur*, when the symptoms are complicated with hæmorrhoids, strictures of the rectum, etc.

Generally, the same medicines will cure the disease that are indicated by the character of the gonorrhœal discharge.

For metastatic gonorrhœa of the rectum, *Pulsatilla*, *Mercurius corrosivus*, and *Tussilago petasites* will be found most efficacious.]

VII. Gonorrhœal arthritis, rheumatism, articular inflammation, swelling of the knee, arthritis blennorrhoica, rheumatismus gonorrhoicus, gonitis gonorrhoica, gonocele, etc.

Gonorrhœal arthritis is one of the sequelæ of gonorrhœa, which was formerly overlooked and is denied even now by many. Its existence is admitted, however, by such men as Astley Cooper, Graves, Simon, Eisenmann, Lawrence, Cumano, Holscher, Rayer, Rostan, Sigmund, Hebra, etc. Even Ricord, who denies the existence of this disease, admits that in persons who are subject to rheumatism, gonorrhœa may induce a gonorrhœal arthritis or rheumatism. Casenave has shown, however, that an articular rheumatism which happens to supervene during gonorrhœa, has to be carefully distinguished from gonorrhœal rheumatism. Articular rheumatism which happens to supervene during the existence of gonorrhœa rarely occurs at a period when gonorrhœal arthritis generally sets in, namely, about the fourth, fifth, or sixth week of gonorrhœa; in most cases the rheumatism is already existing previous to the gonorrhœal infection taking place. In gonorrhœal arthritis the pain is generally seated in the knee, sometimes in the elbow and in the tarsal joint; in rheumatism, on the contrary, every joint, even the muscles, are affected; it is either shifting from joint to joint, or else seated.

Gonorrhœal articular rheumatism is generally located in the knee-joint, and is distinguished from gonorrhœal arthritis by a much more intense reaction which is almost entirely wanting in the latter. Articular rheumatism leaves the gonorrhœal discharge almost entirely unaltered; in gonorrhœal arthritis it is either lessened or suppressed.

With proper treatment the disease lasts from three to four weeks. According to the symptoms, one or more from among the following list of remedies will have to be selected : *Aconite, Bryonia, Mercurius sol., Nux vom., Pulsat., Rhus t., Rhododendron, Sulphur, Tussilago petasites ;* electro-magnetism is an admirable remedy in this disease.

[*Aconite*, if the swelling develops itself suddenly, with all the symptoms of an acute inflammation, intense burning and lancinating or tearing pains, excessive tenderness to the touch, etc.

Bryonia may be substituted for Aconite when the acute stage has subsided, and the pains have moderated; or it may be given in alternation with Aconite.

Mercurius sol. will be found suitable, if the original discharge was of a syphilitic character, or some intensely-acting mercurial preparation may be employed.

Pulsatilla is useful when the knee-joint is the principal seat of the disease, with deep-seated soreness and aching pains in the joints.

Rhus. tox. and *Rhododendron* may be resorted to, if the pains are mitigated by motion, and the inflammatory symptoms are very slight, the swelling is large and hard.]

Gonorrhœal Disorganizations.

I. Chronic Inflammation and Suppuration of the Prostate Gland.

If an acute inflammation of the prostate gland is not speedily scattered,—and it is but too frequently the case that the aid of a physician is only sought when this disease has already reached its acme,—it generally terminates in suppuration, or passes into the chronic form.

Generally the patients first complain of a painful pressure in the perinæum, and which is at first felt only during an emission of urine or semen, but afterwards becomes continuous, and is always worse during the above-mentioned emissions. At a later period the pain increases to a burning, extending to the glans and even downwards to the testicles and thighs. From the urethra an albuminous, colorless, ropy fluid is discharged, which sometimes closes the orifice of the urethra, is secreted more copiously after an emission of semen, urine or after stool, and is particularly increased during a constipated state of the bowels by pressing upon the prostate gland, by excesses in drinking or sexual pleasures, by taking cold or by physical exertions; the pains are likewise aggravated at such periods.

Under the operation of these same causes, the urging to urinate is likewise more violent, the irritation extends to the bladder, the urine is expelled by fits and starts; it is mixed with mucous flocks, the stream is sometimes divided, and a little urine constantly remains behind in the bladder, of a dark color, a pungent ammoniacal odor, and causing an increased irritation of the organ. In order to be sure of a correct diagnosis, the parts should be explored simultaneously with the finger through the rectum, and with the catheter through the urethra. The prostate gland becomes variously disorganised, at times only swollen, at others harder or softer; at times again its tissue is altered, or there are adhesions between the prostate and the surrounding parts.

The existence of suppuration may be inferred from a constant desire to urinate, pain when urinating, and the presence of tenacious mucous and pus in the urine. In such a case, the constitutional irritation is quite considerable; there are frequent chills, febrile motions, and even delirium. In the perinæal region a dull, painful throbbing is experienced.

The suppurative process is either going on in the body of the gland, or in the surrounding cellular tissue.

The abscess generally opens into the urethra; sometimes the discharge is accomplished by means of the catheter. The dangerous symptoms speedily disappear after the discharge of the pus, which is drawn off by the catheter. The pus may likewise discharge into the bladder or rectum. In the former case the pus is expelled together with the urine; in the latter case, blood and pus flow out of the rectum. After the breaking of the abscess, no matter in what direction, the morbid phenomena, especially the retention of urine, subside, and perfect recovery soon takes place.

If the pus cannot be discharged, which takes place in case the substance of the gland is affected, the consequences may be very distressing.

The following remedies will be found the most suitable in chronic inflammation and suppuration of the prostate gland: *Arg. nitr.*, *Aurum*, *Arsen.*, *Acid. nitr.*, *Carbo. anim.*, *Calcar.*, *Capsic.*, *Cannab.*, *Conium*, *Iodine*, *Lycopod.*, *Merc. sol.*, *Nux vom.*, *Pulsat.*, *Rhodod.*, *Sal ammoniacum*, *Silicea*, *Sulphur*, *Spongia*, *Thuja*, *Tussilago petasites* and *Uva ursi.*

[*Thuja* is one of the most efficient remedies for hypertrophy, engorgement and infiltration of the prostate gland, also suppuration; in a case of suppuration of this gland, reported by Trinks, the exhibition of Thuja was followed by an increase of the pains and of the urging to urinate, and by the protrusion of hæmorrhoidal tumors, with violent burning pains; the disease was cured completely and in a short time by the binniodide of potash.

Arsenicum may be resorted to if the patient feels very much debilitated by the disease; if the disease threatens to assume a malignant form, and a foul ichor is discharged from the gland, with fetid colliquative diarrhœa, foul urine, etc.

Mercurius sol., if the urine contains shreds of mucus, or deposits a chalk-like, purulent sediment, and a heavy, aching pain is experienced in the perinæal region. The other mercurial preparations may prove serviceable, if the soluble mercury should fail.

The *biniodide of potash* has been mentioned previously as an important agent in suppuration of the prostate gland.

Iodine may prove serviceable in induration or subsequent atrophy of the gland.

Silicea may be used in chronic suppuration of the gland, with heat and soreness in the gland, discharge of pus with the urine or stool, urging to urinate, costiveness.]

II. Strictures of the Urethra.

By strictures of the urethra we understand a diminution of the transverse diameter of this canal, owing to some morbid alteration of its tissue.

The most frequent cause of strictures of the urethra is gonorrhœa. This form of blennorrhœa, which does not arise from an ulcer, and has the character of a genuine catarrhal inflammation of the mucous membrane of the urethra, yields to proper treatment, even in its most acute forms, in two or three weeks, without leaving a trace behind. After such a treatment the mucous membrane resumes its former elasticity and dilatability, as if no discharge had ever existed.

But most patients, especially young people, are prevented by a feeling of ill-timed modesty, from applying to a trustworthy physician, and prefer submitting to the improper treatment of some quack. The discharge remains uncured, and strictures, inflammations of the kidneys or bladder, are the consequence. If quacking remains inefficient, a physician is applied to. In the meanwhile the inflammation of the mucous membrane becomes chronic, and an exudation takes place in its tissue, in consequence of which the urethra becomes narrower, and the free emission of urine is prevented.

After syphilitic or virulent gonorrhœa strictures of the urethra are quite common. This is owing to the pressure of a syphilitic ulcer in the urethra, from which the pus is discharged. Such ulcers are generally seated on one side of the inner wall of the urethra, and leave a cicatrix even in the most fortunate cases. This cicatriced tissue is constantly disposed to contractions which likewise lead to strictures, but different from those which result from a common gonorrhœal discharge.

Another cause of stricture is the *varicose engorgement* of the blood-vessels of the mucous membrane of the urethra. The engorged vessels form prominences in the urethra, generally in the region of the neck of the bladder, in consequence of which the urethra becomes narrower and the emission of urine is sometimes rendered impossible.

Strictures are sometimes, but less frequently, induced by *tubercles* in the sub-mucous cellular tissue of the urethra. With reference to the above mentioned causes we distinguish *spasmodic*, *organic* or *continuous* and *mixed strictures*.

1. *Spasmodic strictures* are said to result from anomalous contractions of the organic and animal muscular fibres of the urethra. This form of stricture is doubted by some. It is said to occur principally in irritable individuals, hæmorrhoidal subjects, and in persons suffering with chronic inflammation of the prostate gland.

2. *Organic strictures* are the real strictures of the urethra, the treatment of which requires our most particular attention.

This class of strictures has likewise been divided into several varieties, based upon pathological distinctions:

a. Inflammatory strictures, which develope themselves even during the course of an acute gonorrhœa. The mucous membrane is swollen throughout its whole extent, owing to which the space of the urethral canal is diminished and the discharge of urine is less and even entirely prevented. This kind of stricture disappears together with the gonorrhœa under proper treatment.

b. Membraneous strictures, arising from the formation of folds or valves in the mucous membrane.

c. Fleshy strictures, caused by a partial swelling of the lining membrane.

d. Fibrous or cartilaginous strictures, caused by cicatrized wounds, ulcers, fissures, etc.

e. Varicose strictures, arising from engorgement of the blood-vessels coursing along the inner walls of the urethra, especially in the region of the neck of the bladder.

3. By *mixed strictures* we mean such as arise from a spasmodic condition and an organic ulceration of the tissues They may likewise be caused by the insertion of a bougie through a contracted portion of the urethra. Riding on

horseback, forced marches, excessive drinking and venereal abuse may likewise lead to such complications.

As regards *locality*, the whole canal may be constricted so as to form a narrow tube. Spasmodic strictures are always seated in the membranous portion, for this is the only portion of the urethra which is surrounded by muscular fibres.

Organic strictures are most frequently located five or six inches from the internal orifice of the urethra, directly under the symphysis pubis, at the junction of the spongy with the membranous portion. They occur less frequently at the termination of the navicular fossa, or in the prostatic portion.

Let us now pass to the *phenomena* of a stricture. Soon after the termination of an improperly treated gonorrhœa drops of mucus are discharged from the urethra, which are only seen in the morning, when the orifice is found closed with the mucus. The bed-linen and the shirt exhibit dirty yellow stains. This kind of discharge is generally termed "*goutte militaire*," and is not infectious. Such discharges from the urethra always point to incipient strictures.

Another sign by which the existence of stricture is known, is the *thinness of the stream*, always accompanied with an increased slowness of the stream which ceases to form a curve, but comes down in a rather perpendicular direction.

The shape of the stream is likewise altered; first it becomes flat, and finally divides into several branches, which are twisted about one another like a cork-screw. Sometimes the stream scatters all around on leaving the urethra; at last the urine comes off in drops and very slowly.

The urging to urinate is constant, and is particularly troublesome at night. The urine is discharged with great trouble; the patient has to press both his hands upon his knees or upon some other hard object near by; during such efforts the face and neck turn red, tears flow out of the eyes, and in more inveterate cases the patients are sometimes obliged to assume a position, when urinating, as if they would go to stool. If this condition lasts any length of time, hernia and prolapsus of the rectum are apt to take place.

Such efforts are always accompanied by great pain. This pain is of various kinds, prickling, stinging, burning, itching and more or less acute; it excites a sensation of heat, which sometimes increases to a burning, as with a red-hot iron, and is so distressing that the patients refrain from urinating as long as they can in order not to excite the pain. In consequence of being retained in this manner, the urine becomes more acrid, and causes erosions, soreness, rhagades and ulcerations behind the stricture. At first the dysuria is only felt during an emission of urine; after a while it continues even after the emission.

Not only the emission of the urine, but also that of the semen causes pain, which is sometimes so violent that the patients dread sexual intercourse and frequently avoid it altogether. According to the statements of some patients, the pain which is experienced during an emission of semen is more acute than that which an emission of urine causes.

In the course of the disease an inability to retain the urine, or incontinence of urine, sets in. This incontinence may be complete or partial. If partial, a small quantity of urine is discharged involuntarily drop by drop after every urinary emission; the clothes get wet, and, after awhile, a fetid odor is spread in spite of the utmost cleanliness. This dribbling of the urine is caused by a quantity of urine accumulating behind the stricture in a kind of sacculated enlargement, and flowing off through the stricture by its own gravitation. Complete incontinence is much more distressing and inconvenient. In this case the enlargement extends to the neck of the bladder, on which account the bladder is unable to retain the urine which passes off continually and involuntarily. Such unfortunate patients have to wear a receiving vessel fastened to the parts.

The most horrible accompaniment of strictures is *retention of urine*, which really endangers life. Inasmuch as this affection may likewise arise from other causes, we will recur to it in a special section.

The alterations which occur in the quantity and quality of

the urine in strictures, require to be examined. The quantity of the urine does not differ much from that of the urine in a normal state of health. It is lessened if the patients, in order to avoid the necessity of emitting it on account of the great pain, endeavor to diminish the natural quantity of the urine by diminishing the quantity of the beverage which they are in the habit of drinking. This, however, does not diminish the urinary tenesmus; for, owing to the diminution of the quantity of the beverage, the urine becomes more salt and irritating than it was formerly. The urging is more frequent, very painful; stranguary sets in, and the urine is discharged in drops.

The quality of the urine is altered in this, that it contains a greater amount of salt and ammonia than in its healthy condition; it is moreover mixed with pus and mucus; after standing for a time, a cloudy, dirty white precipitate goes down, and a pungent, disagreeable, ammoniacal odor emanates from the urine.

Beside these symptoms, an exploration of the urethra by means of the catheter completes the certainty of our diagnosis as to the existence of a stricture.

This exploration may either be instituted with *inflexible, metallic*, or with *flexible, soft catheters*, termed *bougies*. We omit a description of the mode in which the catheter is to be introduced; physicians may consult surgical works in reference to this subject, and laymen will probably not venture on such an operation, which requires a good deal of dexterity and practical experience. This same remark applies to the various forms and the materials of probes.

We will simply state in this place, that a catheter or bougie is to be introduced, if we desire to find out the number, locality, length, form and condition of the strictures, and that the thickness of the bougie should be proportionate to the size of the stream.

The course of a stricture is very irregular; it may be shortened or prolonged by natural disposition, a suitable mode of life, and by various diseases. The stricture is generally made worse by errors in diet, an exciting mode of life, and by venereal excesses. A stricture never gets well of itself, but is always disposed to terminate in a complete closing of the urethra, and consequent retention of urine. To prevent this result, a seasonable treatment is absolutely necessary.

The *prognosis* is generally doubtful, especially if a suitable treatment is not instituted in season. It likewise depends upon the seat and the condition of the stricture. The nearer it is to the outer portion of the urethra, the more recent, the more dilatable, the less extensive and contracted the stricture, the sooner it is removed. Complications and constitutional derangements increase the difficulty and render the prognosis less favorable.

In regard to *treatment*, I do not think that homœopathic physicians will be able to dispense with mechanical means. Spasmodic strictures can indeed be removed by internal treatment permanently and without pain; likewise other kinds of stricture, provided the disorganization of the mucous membrane is not too far advanced; in such a case the specific remedial virtues of our drugs may yet succeed in effecting a resolution of the morbid alterations of the tissue of the urethra. But if the disorganization has assumed a fibrous character, manual interference is indispensable.

In the treatment of spasmodic strictures, and of the lighter forms of swelling of the mucous membrane of the urethra, the following remedies will be found the most suitable, according as the symptoms may require: *Agaricus*, *Agr. nitr.*, *Argilla*, *Belladonna*, *Bismuth*, *Camphora*, *Clematis*, *Con. mac.*, *Silicea*, *Kali*, *Petrol.*, *Digit.*, *Iodium*, *Nitric acid*, *Opium*, *Stramon.*, *Terebinth*, *Thuja*. (*Cantharides*, *Mercur. sol.* and *Sulph.* should not be omitted.—Ed.)

[The principal remedies for spasmodic strictures, with their symptomatic indications, are:

Aconite: with inflammatory fever; constant and distressing urging to urinate, with inability to pass any urine.

Cantharides: For similar symptoms, with discharge of a few drops of blood instead of urine.

Belladonna: For frequent urging, the urine looking natural or gold-colored, with cerebral congestion, and costiveness.

Camphora: Strangury, burning of the urine, thin stream.

Digitalis: Continual desire to urinate, emitting only a few drops each time, with sensation as if the bladder were too full; or pressing and burning in the middle of the urethra as if too narrow.

Argentum nitricum: Burning urine, pain in the urethra as if swollen and closed.

Nux vomica: Painful, ineffectual desire to urinate.

Opium: Spontaneous interruption of the stream when urinating; or complete suppression of the urinary secretion.

Terebinthina: Dysuria, also complete suppression of urine, also with painful erections.

Thuja: Difficult micturition; the stream is arrested half a dozen times before the urine is entirely voided.]

In organic strictures, a surgical operation is unavoidable. Before, however, resorting to it, we have to distinguish between strictures which allow the urine and the instruments to pass, and such as do not, or only with great difficulty. This second variety will be discussed more fully in the article on retention of urine, section of the diseases of the urinary organs. For the present we will simply mention the various operations which are employed with success for the purpose of effecting the dilatation of the contracted urethra. They are

1. Simple *dilatation;*
2. *Cauterization;* and
3. *Incision.*

1. *Dilatations.*

This method is the one which is most generally employed, and which I likewise prefer, for it has never failed me in my practice which has been pretty extensive. Some employ for this purpose metallic, others flexible bougies. The bougie may either be left in the urethra for a longer period, (permanent dilatation,) or a momentary introduction may suffice (temporary dilatation). I prefer the use of elastic bougies made of caoutchouc and gutta percha.

The size of the bougie should be proportionate to the size of the stream. At first thin bougies should be used, and their size should be gradually increased. Holding the bougie as we do a common writing pen, we cautiously introduce it into the urethra. It may happen that, before reaching the stricture, the bougie is arrested by a fold of the mucous membrane, or by one of the mucous follicles situated along the lower wall of the urethra. In such a case the bougie is to be drawn back, and the penis to be pulled forward for the purpose of removing the obstacle. If the stricture is reached, we endeavour to work the bougie through the narrow opening; if we do not succeed, a thinner bougie has to be tried. We must not lose courage, if we find it hard to overcome the difficulty; with skill and perseverance we shall finally gain our object. If, after passing the bougie into the narrow opening, the obstacle remains nevertheless unconquered, we have to attribute the difficulty to the windings of the stricture. This new obstacle is overcome by turning the bougie irregularly in different directions, until we finally succeed in penetrating the bladder.

In order to be perfectly satisfied whether the bougie has really penetrated the stricture, we hold it quite loosely between the fingers; if the stricture is passed, the bougie will remain in its place; if it is simply bent in the urethra, its elasticity will cause it to bound back again.

If the canal should be very narrow, it is sometimes an advantage to inject sweet almond oil into the urethra.

The bougie may be introduced once or twice a day. At every new trial, the bougie which had been used last, and had been introduced with ease, has to be used again, and to be left five or ten minutes in the urethra, before we replace it by one of larger size.

The length of time during which the bougie should be

allowed to remain in the urethra, depends upon the patient's own feelings. Some bear the presence of the bougie for an hour; very irritable and sensitive persons are frequently made sick, if the bougie is left too long. This sensitiveness decreases however after repeated trials.

At the commencement of the treatment, the bougies should not be changed without great caution. Bougies of larger size should only be used after a considerable dilatation of the stricture has taken place. The operation of the bougie is materially arrested by a few doses of *Belladonna*, *Clematis* or *Thuja*.

After using the bougie and the suitable remedies for about three weeks, the patient is generally cured, and the stricture together with all the diffiulties in voiding urine, removed. However it is not well to discontinue the use of the bougie immediately; on the contrary, it is advisable to continue the use thereof for sometime longer.

In the case of sensitive and irritable persons, who suffer much pain from the introduction of the bougie, one or two days should be allowod to elapse before another introduction of the bougie is attempted, until the parts have become less irritable. If, in spite of all care and trouble, we should not succeed, upon a first trial, in introducing a bougie, were it ever so thin, the introduction of the instrument may be attempted while the patient is in a tepid bath. Sometimes we will find it more easy to introduce a bougie of larger than one of a smaller size.

The dilatation of the urethra by means of a bougie has several advantages. 1st, a mechanical enlargement of the stricture; and 2d, a restoration of the depressed vitality of the urethral mucous membrane, an increased activity of the reproductive system, and consequent absorption of the adventitious growth.

The symptoms are likewise favorably altered by the use of the bougie. Even after its first introduction, the urine is voided with more ease, and the patient is very much relieved.

As the stricture is more dilated, the stream increases in

size, the urine is voided in less time, and the last drops even are properly expelled by the bladder, instead of the former dribbling.

On first introducing the bougie, the mucous discharge is somewhat increased; but it decreases in proportion as the stricture dilates, and finally ceases altogether.

The urging to urinate disappears already after a few trials. This enables the patient to have a quiet rest at night, by which means the general health is improved and the cure facilitated.

The efforts which the patient had to make, in order to void the urine, and the pain which he experienced during micturition or during an embrace, decrease likewise after several introductions of the bougie. The dribbling of the urine, and the ischuria likewise disappear, provided, however, the latter disease did not arise from any other cause.

The urine becomes clearer after awhile; it is no longer mixed with blood and mucus, loses its pungent, ammoniacal odor, and the sediment gradually disappear.

We have to devote a few remarks to *permanent dilatation;* which, though less desirable than the temporary dilatation, may nevertheless be rendered necessary now and then by circumstances. This is particularly necessary when the physician is prevented from seeing his patient every day. For the permanent dilatation we generally use an elastic catheter. The instrument is introduced in the same manner as the bougie, and, after having penetrated the stricture, it is fastened to the abdomen by means of a thin string, and left in this position until the next day, so that it can be easily moved to and fro in the stricture. Next day we use a catheter a little larger in size, and which it is difficult to pass through the stricture. Every second or third day we select a catheter of a somewhat larger size, until the urethra has acquired its normal diameter. The outer orifice of the catheter is closed by means of a little tampon which the patient removes himself when he desires to void urine. If the physician should be unable to see his patient every day, or if the patient should live at a distance, the patient may introduce the bougie himself after being shown how.

2. *Cauterization.*

Without having the least desire to say a word in favor of this method, we do not deem ourselves authorized to omit it, were it for no other reason than because it is not long since it was universally practised. This method of treatment may be traced as far back as Ambrosius Paré, towards the middle of the sixteenth century. Two hundred years after this period it was superseded by the method of dilatation, until revived again by Hunter about the middle of the last century. Ducamp is the one who has most distinguished himself in the treatment of strictures by cauterization. Owing to his efforts and example, it became almost the exclusive method of treatment of strictures of the urethra during a period of ten years from 1820 to 1830. It was soon found, however, that this method did not obviate the liability to relapses caused by the contracting cicatrix. On this account it was opposed by a number of modern physicians, and finally had to give way again to the method of dilatation.

The caustic is applied in the following manner, After having explored the locality and extent of the stricture, the caustic is applied by means of a canula of gum elastic, platina, gold or silver, to the end of which a little capsule of platina filled with liquid nitrate of silver is attached. A rod is riveted to the capsule, by means of which it can be moved to and fro, and turned about. At its extremity, or on the sides, the canula has openings through which the caustic is brought in contact with the stricture. To the canula is attached a graduated scale marked with figures, by which we can ascertain how far the capsule has penetrated in the urethra. The caustic remains in contact with the stricture for half a minute or a whole minute, after which the rod with the capsule, and finally, the whole instrument is withdrawn. On the second and third day, bougies are introduced for the purpose of dilating the canal and facilitating the coming off of the scurf.

This proceeding is repeated every three or four days until the obstacle is entirely removed. To complete the cure, bougies are used in order to secure a proper dilatation of the urethra, and this method is continued until the wound is completely cicatrized.

3. *Scarification, Operations with Cutting Instruments.*

This method is as old as any of the former. Ambrosius Paré likewise resorted to it, and employed for his purpose an instrument which he termed *queue de ret.* Later surgeons employed for this purpose trocarts; Amussat invented an urethratome and scarificators. Modern surgeons, such as Diondi, Dieffenbach, Pauli, Stafford, Tanebon, Despiney, Martial, Duynerris and Ricord, have contrived various instruments for the division of strictures. The most simple instrument is undoubtedly that of Ricord consisting of a tube containing a stiletto with a small blade, which can be pushed out ad libitum.

Before this instrument can be employed, the stricture has to be sufficiently dilated by means of bougies, to admit of the passage of the instrument. The instrument, closed and well oiled, is passed through the stricture, and the stiletto with its blade having been pushed forward, the stricture is divided several times, from before backwards, and from behind forwards. To prevent the premature adhesions of the incisions, bougies have to be introduced. The operation has to be repeated until the difficulty is entirely removed,

On account of the many inconveniences consequent upon this operation, among which the hæmorrhage which sometimes accompanies it, and is sometimes quite considerable, is not by any means one of the least troublesome, it, as well as the treatment by cauterization, has been abandoned by most physicians, so much more as its results are not more promising than those of the method of dilatation. It is only resorted to now-a-days in the case of valvular strictures, or such as are located in the anterior portion of the urethra.

Gonorrhœa of the female, fluor albus, leucorrhœa.

Leucorrhœa is an affection of the female organs analogous to the gonorrhœa of the male, and, by many physicians, is looked upon as a variety of syphilis. This, however, is no more true than that every form of gonorrhæa is a syphilitic disease.

The female organs are much more frequently affected with blennorrhœa than the male, probably because the mucous surface of the former is more extensive, and the inflammatory irritation may invade several organs. On this account four varieties of female gonorrhœa have been adopted: 1, *urethritis*, inflammation of the urethra; 2, *vulvitis*, inflammation of the vulva; 3, *vaginitis*, inflammation of the vagina; 4, *uteritis*, inflammation of the uterus. We will define each of these four varieties more in detail, as soon as the course of female gonorrhœa generally shall have been treated of.

A few days after an impure coït, a heat, burning and drawing are experienced in the parts; the mucous membrane is drier than usual, and very sensitive, and of a dark red color either throughout its whole extent or only in some of its parts. The large, and afterwards the small labia begin to swell. The rubbing of the clothes in walking causes a pain; the pains during micturition are still more distressing, particularly when the last drops flow over the inflamed mucous membrane. Soon after, the patient complains of pains in the small of the back, especially when sitting. A sense of tension, tickling, and very frequently an irresistible desire for an embrace, a real nymphomania set in. Coït is, however, painful. Many women experience, moreover, a languor, a tearing in the extremities, especially in the thighs, and colicky pains. These phenomena generally cease after the appearance of the discharge. This is at first watery, yellowish, turbid, and sometimes mixed with blood, and leaves a grayish stain on the linen. Afterwards the discharge assumes a dark yellow, greenish color, becomes thick, has an offensive smell, and is so copious that it flows down the thigh on walking or rising from a seat. When the inflammation decreases, the discharge becomes whitish, milky, sometimes very thick, cheesy, and flocculent. At first the mucous membrane looks red, and is marked with roundish spots or streaks, which afterwards change to erosions. After the disease has lasted for a time, the follicles begin to swell and become prominent, imparting an uneven and granular feel to the mucous membrane. At the commencement of the menses the pain gets worse, and the discharge increases a good deal. During the menstrual flow, however, the pains abate, and reappear again as before, after the cessation of the menstrual periods.

As regards the causes, and disposition to female gonorrhœa, the remarks we have offered concerning this disease in the male, are likewise applicable to the female. Every cause which is capable of causing an inflammation of the mucous membrane is likewise capable of causing an inflammation with a mucous discharge in the pudendum. The habitual exposure of the female parts to the atmospheric air increases their liability to disease. Hence leucorrhœa may be caused by a variety of influences, and may affect every age. There are even cases where a copious discharge of mucous from the pudendum has been observed in infants during their passage from the womb into the light of day. It frequently happens that girls are attacked with leucorrhœa during the period of dentition, accompanied with considerable pain; also during the course of many eruptive diseases, scrofula, etc.

Blennorrhœa of the pudendum may arise from a variety of irritating causes, from onanism, premature sexual intercourse, especially when the vulva is too small, excessive sexual intercourse, mechanical injuries, foreign bodies in the vagina,* such as the pessary. It is quite common, even among perfectly healthy women, that they should have a leucorrhœal discharge shortly before and shortly after the period. A

* Some time ago I treated a girl of 17 years for leucorrhœa, which had been caused by the girl having rubbed the vagina for a considerable period of time with a carrot, which had been introduced for that purpose into the vagina.

similar discharge takes place during the last weeks of pregnancy and at the critical age when the menses are about to stop. In large cities most women are troubled with leucorrhœa to some extent, which is probably attributable to the weather, to their mode of dressing and living, to excessive reading, to sedentary habits and other circumstances. Coffee with milk is likewise supposed capable of causing leucorrhœa.

Gonorrhœa may likewise be caused by an infectious contagion, without, however, being syphilitic, and without causing chancrous ulcers. In the case of the female it is indeed more difficult than in the case of the male, to ascertain the contemporaneous existence of syphilitic ulcers and the leucorrhœal discharge, hence a mistake is not so very difficult.

The infection of the gonorrhœal contagion generally takes place during coït. It may likewise take place by the female parts being barely touched by the diseased penis. In order to be perfectly certain of the true nature of the discharge in the case of females, it is absolutely necessary to explore the parts by means of a speculum; otherwise the physician might be left in the dark and miss the cure.

Before we proceed to the treatment of leucorrhœa, we will consider each of the four forms of leucorrhœa distinguished with reference to the particular *seat* of the disease.

I. Urethritis.

If the inflammation is located in the urethra, it is first revealed to us by itching, pain, swelling of the orifice of the urethra, urging to urinate. It scarcely ever exists by itself, and is generally accompanied by inflammation of the labia and the vagina. It is readily recognized by the drops of pus which are seen at the orifice of the urethra. Immediately after voiding urine or washing the parts, the traces of the inflammation have to be looked for on the linen which the patients wear on their persons. We see on the shirt small, isolated, opaque spots of a yellowish-green color. In order to be perfectly sure of the character of the disease, we have to institute an examination *per speculum*, and by the touch.

For this purpose the index-finger is introduced into the vagina, and the urethra is compressed from behind forwards and upwards, by which means a yellowish, thick mucus is pressed out of the orifice of the urethra.

II. Vulvitis.

This inflammation is recognized even after a superficial examination of the parts, and is the same as the balanorrhœa of the male. If the inflammation is very acute, the swelling of the labia sometimes encroaches upon the orifice of the vagina. The small labia are œdematous; they constitute a thick, bluish-red, shining, disk-shaped swelling, and are covered with a number of erosions; likewise the clitoris and its surrounding parts. The labia majora are tense, dark-red and very prominent. The contact of the urine causes much pain, and the introduction of the speculum is impossible. The follicles are swollen, and constitute more or less considerable prominences which sometimes terminate in suppuration, constituting the so-called *abscessus pudendi*. When the labia are intensely inflamed, the warmth of the bed becomes intolerable, fever sets in, and the patient is tormented by thirst and sleeplessness. On examining the parts, we discover a viscid, purulent fluid of a specific odor, which sometimes dries up in the hair of the pudendum, forming a thick, crusty covering. Sometimes this secretion is so acrid that the external surface of the labia majora, the perinæum, anus, and even the thighs become inflamed, excoriated, and likewise secrete a purulent fluid.

Corpulent women are particularly predisposed to this kind of leucorrhœa. Such patients find it troublesome to walk; their sexual instinct is generally more active, but the sexual act itself is painful. In the case of little girls, leucorrhœa is either the result of some internal disease, or more frequently of mechanical injuries, touching, rape. Andrieux de Brionde states that newly-married women frequently experience stinging pains in the pudendum the first days after their marriage, which he attributes to an unusual desire for sexual intercourse.

Onanism is a frequent cause of the disease. As long as this vice is indulged in, the disease will of course continue. The most careful watching, the most serious exhortations, even punishment, are frequently insufficient to stop this vile practice. Durand Tarvel relates the case of a girl of nine years whose clitoris was removed by the knife, in order to stop this destructive habit. The operation was very painful. In order to arrest the hæmorrhage, the actual cautery was applied; but scarcely had the wound been healed when the child resumed its former habits.

III. Vaginitis. Inflammation of the Vagina.

This disease is more frequent than inflammations of the external parts. It is generally accompanied with blennorrhœa of the labia. The inflammation is either seated in the superficial mucous membrane, or in the mucous follicles or bursæ; if very acute, the whole substance of the mucous membrane and the subjacent sub-mucous cellular tissue may be invaded.

In such a case women sometimes complain of pain in the pelvis, heat, and sense of weight in this region; intense heat in the vagina, pains which frequently strike to the renal regions; all these symptoms are worse during a walk, at stool, and when voiding the urine. The sexual desire is generally more intense, and may be gratified without pain, provided the inflammation is not too acute. The mucus is discharged in quantities. Either the whole vagina or only a portion thereof may be affected. If the follicles are principally invaded, we distinguish a number of miliary granulations with the finger. In every case of this kind the mucous membrane is redder than usual, partially denuded of its epithelium, and covered with small, superficial ulcers. A mucus which is frequently mixed with blood, and pus are secreted; this secretion has an acid reaction, and leaves yellow or yellowish green spots on the linen.

IV. Uteritis. Inflammation of the Uterus.

The catarrhal inflammation of the uterus is the most obstinate form of leucorrhœa, and the most distressing in its consequences. It is accompanied with considerable derangements of the menstrual functions, violent hæmorrhages, difficult conception, degeneration of the fetus, disposition to miscarriage, and even complete sterility and obliteration of the Fallopian tubes, as is frequently observed in prostitutes. This inflammation is recognized by redness and dryness of the neck of the uterus. The neck is covered with a whitish, thick, adhering mucus, secreted from the internal orifice of the womb or from all the surrounding parts. The patients complain of heaviness and drawing in the pelvis and small of the back, and, on sitting down, frequently experience a burning pain. Erosions soon develope themselves round the os tincæ, with superficial, uneven ulcerations, which are covered here and there with whitish patches of dead epithelium. Sometimes, and particularly in the case of prostitutes who do a large business, inflammation spreads to the inner surface of the uterus, the Fallopiant ubes, the ovaries and the peritonæum; in such a case life may be endangered by the inflammation.

In treating female gonorrhœa homœopathically, we have to consider the seat and extent of the disease, the accessory symptoms which happen to accompany it, and the general condition of the patient. Accordingly, we may have to use one or more of the subsequent list of medicines, either alone or in alternation, or several medicines in a successive series; the selection of the remedy will of course depend upon the symptoms and state of the disease. We will relate these remedies in alphabetical order, and mention the group of symptoms to which each medicine is specifically adapted.

Acid. nitr.: Flat ulcers in the vagina as if covered with a yellow pus; with a burning, itching pain and leucorrhœa. Discharge of a flesh-colored mucus from the vagina. Swelling at one side of the vagina. (This remedy is particularly adapted to chronic vaginitis.)

Acidum phosphor.: Leucorrhœa before and after the menses, with burning in the urethra.

Acidum sulphur.: Milky, transparent leucorrhœa, painless, but sometimes smarting and mixed with blood, acrid, copious and erosive.

Aconitum: Leucorrhœa, with slight tingling in the parts which is not disagreeable.

Arsenicum: Smarting, gnawing leucorrhœa, causing a soreness of the parts with which it comes in contact; when standing the discharge drops down, accompanied with emission of flatulence. Redness of the parts.

Aurum: Profuse leucorrhœa which excoriates the perinæum, and the internal sides of the thighs, with vesicular eruption on the parts and back, labor-like pains in the abdomen as if the menses would make their appearance.

Belladonna: Violent dragging towards the sexual parts as if every thing would issue from the abdomen, worse when walking and sitting bent; she feels easier when sitting erect. Bloating of the abdomen, followed by contraction of the same, and by discharge of white mucus from the vagina, violent stitches in the pubic region and the inner parts, at every step she makes, (vaginitis.)

Bryonia: Black, hard pustule on the swollen labium. Swelling of the labia majora. Increase of the discharge which had been decreasing, (vulvitis.)

Calcarea: Burning, jerking leucorrhœa previous to the menses, flowing out like milk. Smarting between the genital organs and thighs. Pressure in the vagina, and tubercles on the labium.

Cannabis: Cutting between the labia during micturition. The orifice of the urethra is closed with a drop of pus. Violent sexual desire with swelling of the vagina. The discharge causes a smarting of the parts which it touches, (urethritis.)

Cantharides: Copious, debilitating leucorrhœa, with pains in the kidneys and a distressing feeling in the pelvis, accompanied with a languid, sallow complexion, depression of spirits, swelling of the neck of the uterus. Burning and itching of the pudendum, (chronic uteritis.)

Chamomilla: Yellow, smarting leucorrhœa from the vagina. Acrid, smarting, watery discharge from the vagina, with smarting, burning as if the parts were excoriated.

Crocus: Leucorrhœa accompanied by paroxysms of acute stitches from the pudendum to the right thigh, as if a knife were thrust into these parts every now and then, suddenly, gradually penetrating into the parts, and with increasing pain.

Graphites: Profuse leucorrhœa in the vagina and painful pressing towards the pudendum.

Ignatia: Violent crampy pressure in the uterus, followed by purulent, corrosive leucorrhœa. Chronic leucorrhœa with excited sexual desire. Swelling of the clitoris with weakness of the remaining portion of the pudendum; coolness of the body, and uterine spasms. (Chronic uteritis.)

Kreasotum: Bloody, flesh-colored, yellow or yellowish-white, leucorrhœa, having a foul smell, especially early in the morning, after rising. Acrid discharge, with itching of the pudendum; jerking, smarting pain in the external parts, and weakness of the legs. (Vagina, &c.)

Lamium: Copious leucorrhœa, coming off in drops, with smarting in the pudendum.

Lycopodium: Copious, bloody or milky leucorrhœa, coming off in paroxysms, worse before the full moon, with burning in the vagina. (Vaginitis.)

Mercurius solubilis: Mild leucorrhœa, of a pale, yellow color, and a sickly, sweetish odor. Discharge of flocks, pus and mucus, of the size of hazle nuts. Purulent leucorrhœa, which does not drop, of a green color, causing a smarting in the anterior portions of the pudendum, which obliges the patient to scratch, especially in the evening and at night; the scratching is followed by a violent burning. Corrosive leucorrhœa with long, lasting itching of the labia, especially shortly before the menses. Pressing in the pudendum, after which the patient has to void a quantity of urine. Swelling of the follicles of the labia. Swelling and inflammation of the internal vagina, as if raw and sore. (Vaginitis and vulvitis.)

Mezereum: Albuminous leucorrhœa. Mucous discharge from the urethra and vagina.

Natrum muriaticum: Greenish leucorrhœa, passing off profusely during a walk, with itching of the pudendum; the discharge is preceded by contractive colic, and a pressing downwards. Aversion to an embrace. Discharge of blood after an embrace, followed by a feeling of ease, and finally, irritable and peevish mood. Painful pressing towards the pudendum.

Nux vomica: Painless discharge of yellow mucus from the vagina. Discharge of fetid mucus from the vagina. Burning in the pudendum, with violent sexual desire. Gnawing, itching eruption on the pudendum. Swelling of the inner vagina, with burning pain, rendering contact intolerable. (Vaginitis.)

Phosphorus: Leucorrhœa with stitches from the vagina to the uterus. Aversion to coït. Leucorrhœa instead of the menstrual discharge; milky leucorrhœa early in the morning when walking. (Uteritis.)

Platina: Leucorrhœa, with pinching in the abdomen, followed by pressing downwards in both groins, alternated by pressure in the pudendum, and increased discharge of blood. Painless, not disagreeable pressure in the lower portion of the pudendum, preceded by a voluptuous tingling in the parts. Painless sensitiveness, and continual pressure in the inner parts, and in the region of the mons veneris, accompanied with an almost unceasing internal chill, and feeling of coldness externally to the hands. Gnawing soreness, as if excoriated, on the left side of, and near the pudendum. Voluptuous tingling in the pudendum, accompanied by a similar, though less perceptible sensation; oppressive anxiety and palpitation of the heart, followed by a painless, not disagreeable pressure in the pudendum, with a languid feeling, and stitches in the fore part of the head. (Uteritis.)

Pulsatilla: Painless leucorrhœa; discharge of a thickish

milk-colored mucus, which is especially perceptible on lying down. Milky leucorrhœa with swelling of the labia. Leucorrhœa with burning pain. Acrid, thin leucorrhœa. Burning, stinging pain in the labia and vagina. Cutting pain at the os tinçæ. (Vaginitis.)

Sabina: Discharge of mucus and blood from the vagina, with labor-like pains. Sharp stitches in the posterior portion of the vagina. Habitual leucorrhœa of the consistence of starch, yellowish, ichorous, fetid, accompanied with painful discharge of blood, almost every fortnight, having a foul smell like old serum. Copious, milky leucorrhœa, causing an itching. Itching of the sexual organs. Increased sexual delight during coït. Discharge of blood between the periods, with sexual excitement. (Vaginitis and vulvitis.)

Sepia: Leucorrhœa, with itching in the vagina. Watery leucorrhœa. Discharge of blood after an embrace, or only when walking. Itching of the pudendum.

Stannum: Discharge of transparent mucus from the vagina, with smarting.

Mercurius corrosivus: Pale-yellow discharge from the vagina, of a nauseous sweetish smell. Pressure at the os tinçæ during coït.

Sulphur: Profuse leucorrhœa. Smarting, burning, thin leucorrhœa, especially early in the morning after rising. Yellow, excoriating discharge from the vagina, accompanied with palpitation of the heart and heat in the face during motion, and followed by burning in the abdomen. Burning of the external pudendum, accompanied by blisters. Violent itching of the clitoris.

Thuja: Leucorrhœa from one period to the other; it is mild and leaves yellowish-green stains on the linen. Mucous discharge from the urethra. Contractive and pressing pain in the pudendum when sitting or rising from a seat. Smarting pain in the pudendum as if the parts were sore, especially during micturition. Stinging in the pudendum when walking. Whitish ulcer on the inside of the labia majora, first causing a pain as if sore when touching it, afterwards itching.

Swelling of both labia, with burning pain only when walking or touching the parts. Smarting and itching of the pudendum, principally in the urethra when voiding urine, and even afterwards. (Urethritis and vulvitis.)

Zincum: Discharge of thick mucus, especially after stool. Constant yawning, with pinching in the abdomen previous to the discharge. Excited sexual desire, especially at night, without lascivious dreams. Terrible desire for self-gratification.

True Venereal or Syphilitic Diseases.

The essence of syphilitic diseases is as yet little known. Pathologically we know that in its first stages it is an inflammation of certain parts of the skin or mucous membrane, which runs a course strikingly analogous to the phenomena caused by violent animal poisons, such as the poison of small pox, dead bodies, etc.

We have already stated that the first symptoms of syphilitic inflammation develope themselves at the spot where the infectious matter is first communicated to the organism.

This inflammation consists in an inflammation of the follicles, and in ulcerations from which a lardaceous, contagious matter is secreted. At this stage the disease yields readily to proper treatment. If the parts round the ulcer have already become hard, it is scarcely possible to avoid a constitutional disease. Afterwards the inflammation spreads to the next lymphatic vessel and to the glands appertaining thereto, and in some cases, produces a poisonous and infectious secretion, even in these parts. This is the commencement of constitutional syphilis, characterised by specific inflammations of the mucous membrane and the dermis in remote parts, and, although no longer capable of producing contagious matter, yet still transmissible to the succeeding generation in congenital syphilis. This is Ricord's view. But Sigmund, of Vienna, and Waller, of Prague, have shown that secondary syphilis is still able to infect others, and to develope in them analogous phenomena. It is only at a later period that the syphilitic disease recedes from the dermis and from the mucous membrane, and, under the form of tertiary syphilis, invades the inner tissues, the fibrous membranes and bones, where it manifests itself in the stage of lentescent inflammations, generally in a circumscribed space, in the shape of nodes, nodous excrescences, tophi, etc., forming peculiar and characteristic, but not contagious morbid products.

Accordingly, considering the internal essence of syphilis, we distinguish two forms of this disease, 1, *primary syphilis*, or the local inflammation produced by the first and direct action of the contagious; and, 2, *constitutional syphilis*, where the whole organism is under the influence of the syphilitic miasm, and of which we again distinguish two forms: A, *secondary*, and B, *tertiary syphilis*.

Primary Syphilis.

Most frequently the syphilitic poison is communicated during coït, by the contact of a sound part with one that is diseased. The infection takes place so much more readily as, during this sexual orgasm, the secretion of the contagious matter, and its absorption by the healthy organs, are considerably increased. In the majority of cases the primary inflammation affects the mucous membranes of the sexual organs, anus, mouth and nipples. It may likewise occur in the eye or nose, in consequence of syphilitic pus getting accidentally to these parts. The syphilitic poison may likewise be transmitted to excoriated parts, wounds or sloughs. Syphilitic ulcerations are frequently seen in small wounds on the fingers, which happened to touch the diseased organs of the same individual. Infection may take place in dressing syphilitic ulcers or during a surgical operation. Sometimes the syphilitic disease is communicated to the infant by the nursing mother, and vice versa. It may likewise be communicated during the passage of the child through the vagina, or by kissing a person, although in the latter case, the mouth or tongue had generally been infected by being applied directly to the diseased organs. The infectious matter may likewise be transmitted by means of tumblers, glasses, spoons, tobacco-pipes, syringes, surgical instruments, lancets, water-closets, etc. Prostitutes who do a large business, sometimes communicate the disease without being themselves affected. The poisonous matter commingles with the vaginal mucus, without infecting them, but is transmitted to the next healthy customer. By washing herself, the girl, whose vaginal mucous membrane had become thick and hardened by excessive use, remains free from the disease.

The principal forms of the primary syphilitic disease are the *primary ulcer* or *chancre*, and the *primarg inflammation of the lymphatic vessels and glands in the neighborhood of the chancre.*

Chancre.

From three to eight days after an impure coït or after contagion has taken place, an itching and slight burning are experienced at the spot where infection had taken place, after which a small red spot comes out, upon which a clear vesicle of the size of a pin's head starts up, whose contents become turbid and purulent. This vesicle breaks and gives place to a small ulcer, with sharp, inverted edges; the opening of the ulcer is narrower than its base. The place where the ulcer is seated, is somewhat hard and swollen. The pus is grayish, bloody, and mixed up with remnants of tissue. Sometimes the patients are not aware of the trouble until after the disease is completely developed. This is particularly the case with men who have a contracted prepuce, and still more with women in whom the infection first took place in the vagina. A chancre may possibly develope itself on any part of the body; it is most frequently seated under the glans, by the frænulum, round the corona glandis, on the inner surface of the prepuce, on the scrotum and at the anus, less frequently in the urethra. According to Professor Sigmund's statement in the Vienna Mediz. Wochenschrift of the 12th of April, 1853, chancres in the urethra are not near as uncommon as has been supposed. Among 483 chancres, 47 were located in the urethra. Chancres are likewise seen on the lips, tongue, eye-lids, ears and fingers; in the female, on the labia, at the entrance of the vagina, in the interior of the vagina, at the neck of the uterus, anus, less frequently at the nipples, lips, tongue, or in the buccal cavity.

Taking the physiological and pathological character of the chancre as a guide, we distinguish the *superficial*, *indurated* and *phagedenic primary syphilitic ulcer*.

The superficial chancre is confined to the upper layer of the skin, only a very small portion of its tissue being destroyed, and the exudation round about being either entirely wanting or only very trifling.

The indurated or so-called Hunterian chancre penetrates through the whole thickness of the skin, the loss of substance is quite considerable, and a quantity of matter is secreted from the ulcer, which becomes rapidly organized and forms all around the ulcer a hard node that can be felt with the finger and constitutes the principal characteristic of this variety of the disease. It is this variety of chancre which is always present in constitutional syphilis.

The phagedenic or diphtheritic chancre is principally developed in impoverished individuals who are at the same time affected with scrofula. The ulcer is covered with a thick gray layer of false membranes, beneath which the destruction of the tissues in surface and depth goes on quite rapidly; the margins are thin, violet, brown, shaggy, rolled up; the secretion is thin, fetid; the cicatrization takes place much more slowly, sometimes not till the ulcerative process has destroyed a considerable extent of tissue by suppuration, both on the surface and in depth; in some cases dangerous hæmorrhage even takes place. The phagedenic ulcer is generally very painful; on the other hand, the constitutional symptoms are very rare, because the poison seems to have exhausted its action by the violence of the local symptoms. Supervening buboes, if ending in suppuration, are disposed to assume the same character as the chancre.

In some cases the chancre becomes gangrenous. In such a case the destruction of the tissues goes on at a rapid rate, so that the whole glans is sometimes destroyed in a short period. After the sloughing a simple ulcer remains which is easily healed.

The treatment must be conformable to the form of the ulcer. Whereas a simple chancre is sometimes cured in from two to three weeks without any signs of constitutional syphilis, the indurated chancre, even under the most careful allopathic treatment, never gets well without symptoms of constitutional syphilis supervening after five or six weeks of treatment. Under homœopathic treatment, which may last from six to eight weeks before a cure is perfected, the constitutional disease is generally prevented. The treatment has to be continued until every trace of induration has disappeared. The ulcer frequently heals without the induration having been entirely removed round the cicatrix; if this is not accomplished to the last vestige, constitutional syphilis will pretty certainly develope itself.

The treatment of the phagedenic chancre has likewise to be continued for some time.

In any variety of chancre the internal treatment has to be accompanied with the utmost cleanliness. The ulcer should be kept covered with lint dipped in water, and should be repeatedly cleansed during the day. A linen rag moistened with cold water may be placed on the ulcer, and the penis wrapt up in a linen bandage. Moreover, the penis should be supported by a suspensory, to prevent the pressure of the blood, by which the cure would be retarded.

Among the remedies to be employed for the cure of chancre, I mention particularly *Acidum nitricum,* the specific effect of which has scarcely ever disappointed me. I have found it particularly indicated by the following conditions: chancres of the orifice of the urethra, prepuce, margin of the prepuce; chancres with bloody, fetid, ichorous pus; small chancres without inflamed borders, with flat edges; considerable swelling of the glans, of the meatus urinarius, which are of a dark-red color and puffed up; small vesicles in the meatus, on the inner surface and margin of the prepuce, which soon break, suppurate and form chancres; deep ulcer at the corona glandis, with elevated, lead-colored, extremely sensitive edges; flat little ulcers at the corona glandis, which look clean, but secrete a strong-smelling matter; itching of the prepuce and damp places on its inner surface; burning of the inflamed and swollen prepuce, the inside of which is denuded of the epidermis and covered with small little ulcers, secreting an ichor that has a pungent, nauseous odor, and stains the linen like bloody pus; simple flat chancre in the vagina, it is covered with yellow pus and burns and itches; and lastly, inflammation of the vagina and labia majora.

Accordingly, *Acidum nitricum* will be found particularly adapted to simple chancre, chancre in the meatus urinarius and in the vagina.

Arsenicum: Gangrenous ulcers with bloody edges, corrosive pus; ulcers with copious secretion of watery, fetid ichor; painless ulcers with hard edges; lardaceous, stinging chancrous ulcers with white places in the middle of the ulcer; Gangrenous chancre on the glans and prepuce; sudden gangrène of the penis.

Accordingly Arsenicum will be found adapted to phagedenic, gangrenous chancres, and accordingly to the indurated chancre of Hunter.

Argentum nitricum: Little ulcers on the prepuce, the tips of which are at first covered with pus, and which gradually spread in extent and become covered with a tallowy or lardaceous substance; swelling and knotty hardness of the urethra, inflammation and pains in the urethra, priapism, dysuria, hæmaturia. (Chancre in the urethra.)

Aurum muriaticum: Chancres of the scrotum, with fetid, ichorous pus.

Calcarea carbon: Chancres on the lower surface of the penis; chancres with burning pain, having the form of rhagades.

Carbo veg.: Readily bleeding chancres with secretion of ichor.

Causticum: Chancres with acrid, corrosive pus or a watery, greenish secretion, with jerking pain, developed out of little blisters, complicated with gout, scurvy and cutaneous eruptions, disposition to fungous formations. (Phagedenic chancre.)

Hepar sulphuris: Readily bleeding chancres with lardaceous edges and fetid secretion.

Iodine: Florid chancres with raised edges that are more or less shaggy, watery secretion.

Mercurius solubilis: Red chancre on the prepuce; spreading and deeply penetrating ulcers on the glans and prepuce; pale-red vesicles on the glans and prepuce, forming small ulcers after breaking; readily bleeding chancres; distressingly painful chancres, secreting a quantity of yellowish-white fetid pus; small chancres with a cheesy bottom, inverted, red edges; inflamed round chancrous ulcers with swelling of the vagina; chancres with edges resembling raw flesh; not very painful ulcers, sensitive to the contact of linen; vesicles at the forepart and on the side of the glans, spreading and penetrating more and more; ulcers of the glans and prepuce with cheesy, lardaceous bottom and hard edges; a number of small red vesicles at the tip of the glans behind the prepuce, breaking after a fortnight and forming little ulcers, which secrete a strong-smelling, yellowish-white matter that stains the linen; afterwards the larger ulcers bleed and are painful when touched, from which the whole body was sympathetically affected; they were round, their edges looked raw and the bottom of the ulcers was covered with a cheesy matter.

Mercurius corrosivus: Chancres with ichor adhering to the bottom of the ulcer so firmly that it cannot be removed by washing; ulcers with thin pus, leaving stains upon the linen as from melted tallow.

Staphysagria: Smarting vesicles on the inside of the labia majora, painful when touched; chancres with fetid ichor.

Sulphur: Chancres with lardaceous white spots and secretion of fetid ichor; ulcers covered with scurfs, and looking like itch-sores; chancres on the prepuce, resembling excoriations; superficial chancres as if the skin were excoriated; red ulcers with lardaceous bottom here and there, lined with a thin matter that can be easily removed; violently itching ulcers, impeding one's walk; torpid ulcers complicated with scrofula, scurvy, gout and cutaneous eruptions.

Thuja: Vesicles on the glans; erosions on the inner surface of the prepuce, which secrete a humor and suppurate; red spots on the prepuce; granular spots on the outer surface of the prepuce, which change to ulcers, become covered with scurfs, itch and burn; pustules on the inside of the prepuce, depressed in the centre, secreting a humor and suppurating, painful only when touched. Burning pain at the corona glandis: flat, itching ulcers surrounded with redness, with stinging pain and unclean bottom. Whitish chancres with hard edges. Chancres with shaggy edges and lardaceous bottom. Chancres with sharply circumscribed edges, and clean, flesh-colored bottom. Chancres with thin, fetid ichor.

During the treatment of primary syphilitic ulcers, the diet should be strictly conformable to the principles of homœopathic practice. Impoverished individuals afflicted with phagedenic chancres, have to use a nutritious diet. Cleanliness is indispensable in every case.

Primary Inflammation of the Neighboring Glands. Buboes.

The inflammation and suppuration of lymphatic glands is generally the first symptom of the infection of the general organism by the syphilitic poison. The inguinal glands, with the surrounding cellular tissue, are generally those that first become affected, inflamed, indurated and then pass into the stage of suppuration. Such swellings are termed *buboes*. They generally arise from the contagious pus of the primary ulcer being absorbed by the lymphatic vessels. One or more, even four weeks generally elapse before the bubo begins to develope itself, sometimes after the chancre is healed. Buboes in the groin occur most frequently when the chancre is seated at the orifice of the urethra or on the frænulum. They likewise accompany chancres seated on the scrotum, external pudendum, in the vagina, on the neck of the uterus, on the mons veneris, on the inner and upper surface of the thighs, on the nates and rectum. Buboes occur rarely in both groins at the same time; this only takes place when chancres exist on both sides of the penis.

Primary ulcers of the lower lip and of the tongue give sometimes rise to buboes under the chin, generally in the corner of the jaw; chancres on the upper lip give rise to buboes at the same place, or in front of the ear; chancres of the wings of the nose and eye-lids, have buboes directly in front of the meatus auditorius externus, at the place where the lobule adjoins it, in some cases above the malar bone; chancres of the nipples give rise to swellings of the axilliary glands; chancres on the fingers result in glandular swellings on the inner side of the elbow joint, and in the axilla.

The cause of primary not constitutional buboes is, as we said before, the absorption of the pus secreted from the primary ulcer. Such buboes develope themselves much more readily and frequently when the primary affection is slight; the secretion of pus is scanty and the inflammation not very acute. The development of the bubo does not depend upon the size of the chancre.

A swelling of the inguinal glands may be induced by external causes, such as a cold, violent or fatiguing exertions of the lower extremities during work or by excessive walking, dancing, etc. Persons who have to stand a good deal, are likewise liable to the development of buboes. They may likewise arise from an excessive enjoyment of sexual intercourse, from errors in diet. Women are generally less liable to buboes than men.

If buboes and chancres co-exist, the invasion of constitutional syphilis may be pretty certainly depended upon. This is probably the reason why buboes are regarded by many physicians as signs of constitutional syphilis.

We distinguish three forms of the primary bubo, corresponding somewhat to the three varieties of chancre; *acute*, inflamed buboes, which generally terminate in suppuration, after which the pus escapes from under the skin; *indolent* or indurated buboes running a long course, and characterized by organized exudations, which do not readily suppurate, and *phagedenic buboes*.

These three varieties of buboes only correspond to the three forms of chancre in so far as this, that they run a similar course; but they are not necessarily related in this manner that indurated buboes accompany indurated chancres, or phagedenic buboes phagedenic chancres. Any variety of bubo may supervene with any form of chancre.

The acute bubo sets in with symptoms of very violent inflammation; the pain and the swelling of the glands increase very rapidly. The surrounding cellular tissue becomes infiltrated with the inflammatory exudation, forming a large and hard wall around the immovable gland. Shortly after, the skin over the tumour becomes hot, a slight redness developes itself in the middle, it becomes shining and very sensitive. The motion of the lower limb is very painful, and the patients frequently complain of a tearing and stitching pain in the whole thigh of the affected side. If the bubo is not scattered, the suppurative process first developes itself in the cellular tissue round the gland. The pus which developes itself round the tumor, gives rise to an oval, soft swelling, in the centre of the tumour; the gland itself still continues to remain hard. Afterwards the suppuration likewise invades the gland. When the tumour is on the point of breaking the skin becomes pale, of a bluish-red color. A violent inflammation of the inguinal glands is sometimes accompanied by œdema of the labia majora, or in both sexes by œdema of the abdomen and of the internal surface of the thighs. Generally fever supervenes, the patients complain of pain in the extremities, coated tongue, full and hard pulse, headache, thirst, etc. When the pus begins to form, chills seti n. If the suppuration is completed, the fever abates, the pains grow less, and the motions of the limb become less painful. The pus escapes in one or more places, generally where the skin is thinnest, nearest the centre. The openings have shaggy, red margins. The pus is of the consistence of cream, and has a greenish, or dark yellow color.

The indolent bubo appears as frequently after primary, particularly after indurated chancres, as after constitutional chancres arising from mucous tubercles (*plagues muqueuses*). This bubo runs a characteristically slow course, and does not begin to grow until the chancre is healed. This growth takes place very slowly; the bubo is very little painful, and feels hard. The skin over the swelling is not altered either in color or temperature; it is moveable over the rugged tumour. When quiet the patients are without pain; it is only when walking or sitting with the thighs considerably bent, or when pressing upon the tumour, that a tension and drawing are experienced. These buboes are much larger than the former variety, and frequently remain unaltered for months, especially in the case of men. Signs of an increased vital action in the tumor develope themselves very slowly. The skin becomes hot and the patients experience slight stitches. The suppurative process, however, only takes place in a portion of the glandular tumor. Small, soft places corresponding to the single glands, and, with an indistinct fluctuation, gradually make their appearance; the skin over these parts is at first of a bright-red color, which afterwards, but slowly, changes to a blue-red. If the tumor breaks in such a place, only a small quantity of thin, flocculent pus is discharged. The opening seldom increases to any great extent; it looks like an unequal, corroded ulcer of the size of a bean, with a dark-yellow, or gray-red rugged bottom; the skin is undermined much farther, but is thinner only round the edges; only a small quantity of a thin yellowish fluid escapes. It scarely ever happens that the entire glands are changed to pus; at the bottom of the ulcer they generally constitute an uneven surface traversed by ridges. Between and by the side of the glands fistulæ with indurated edges develope themselves in various directions, and frequently lead to the secretion of considerable quantities of pus.

The *phagedenic bubo*, as soon as it assumes the condition of an ulcer, has the same properties in regard to shape, spreading and healing, as the phagedenic chancre. It developes itself just as frequently after indurated chancre, as in consequence of the simple spread of the disorganizing phagedenic chancre. The external and internal causes of the phagedenic bubo are the same as those of the phagedenic chancre. It commences with a violent, erysipelatous inflammation of the skin, which spreads rapidly both in extent and depth. The patients complain of violent pain in the tumor, acute fever, the pulse is small and rapid, thirst intense, tongue coated, there is restlessness and sleeplessness. The skin over the tumor soon assumes a livid or dirty-yellow, brown color, becomes gangrenous, sloughs, and the phagadenic chancre is completely developed.

In regard to the syphilitic bubo, we have to observe three things: 1st, to prevent its development (prophylactic treatment); 2d. Scattering the existing tumor; 3d. Healing of the ulcer after suppuration has set in and a discharge of pus has taken place.

The prophylactic treatment implies, 1st, as rapid a cure as possible of the primary chancre; 2d, prevention of the breaking out of new chancres in the neighborhood of the former; 3d, perfect rest of the diseased parts.

The two other conditions of the treatment are met by one or more of the following remedies, which have to be chosen in accordance with the symptoms: *Calcar. carb.*, *Clematis*, *Copaiv.*, *Dulcam.*, *Graphites*, *Kali carb.*, *Lycopod.*, *Merc. sol.*, *Natr. carbon.*, *Nat. mur.*, *Nitric acid.*, *Nux vom.*, *Phosphor.*, *Phosphoric acid*, *Pulsatilla*, *Sulphur*, *Terebinth.*, *Thuja.*

(The principal remedies for buboes are: *Mercurius sol.*, *Kali hydriodicum*, *Silicea*, *Calcarea carb.*, *Acidum nitricum*, *Graphites*, *Thuja.*

Mercurius sol. may be used as soon as the bubo begins

to form; if it should not suffice to prevent the development of the bubo, we may resort to

Kali hydriodicum, which may also be used alternately with Mercurius.

Calcarea and Graphites are suitable for chronic buboes, of a torpid character.

Acidum nitricum, if Mercurius had remained ineffectual, the bubo continues to increase in size, and there is danger of suppuration setting in.

Thuja may be useful, if the syphilitic symptoms were mixed up with condylomatous excrescences on the penis or round the anus.)

This last named remedy is particularly indicated in incipient inflammation of the inguinal glands, characterized by stitching, drawing and tension in the groin, and slight swelling of the inguinal glands. For *indolent buboes*, *Acid. phosphor.*, *Arsen.*, *Con. macul.*, *Ignat.* and *Sepia* have been found most efficacious.

Constitutional Syphilis.

This disease developes itself sooner or later after the appearance of the chancre and the absorption of the syphilitic poison by the organism.

The first signs of constitutional syphilis generally make their appearance some six weeks after the first breaking out of the primary chancre in the shape of syphilitic cutaneous eruptions which are sometimes accompanied by ulceration of the tonsils and mucous membrane of the fauces, or even by syphilitic bone-pains. At a later period ulceration of the laryngeal and nasal mucous membrane supervene.

After the poison has been absorbed by the constitution, its contagious properties are gradually diminished and disappear entirely after the constitutional disease is fully developed. In general, in proportion as the syphilitic disease penetrates the organism, its original character frequently becomes altered to such an extent that it is frequently exceedingly difficult to diagnose the disease and to distinguish it from other equally penetrating disorganizing diseases, such as scrofulosis, tuberculosis, etc.

It does not always follow that primary syphilis must necessarily be followed by the constitutional disease. According to statistical results, among a hundred males affected with disease, from 25 to 48 become constitutionally diseased; and among a hundred females, from 45 to 55. Moreover, the longer and the more copious the secretion of pus from the primary chancre, the more certain is the constitutional disease.

Climate and season have considerable influence on the development of constitutional syphilis. In the temperate zone it is a general rule that the syphilitic eruptions are most frequent during the extremes of temperature, extreme cold or extreme heat. In the damp and cold season, particularly in spring and late in the fall, affections of the buccal and pharyngeal mucous membrane are most frequent. Cold, derangements of the cutaneous action, changes of the weather, damp swellings, etc., favor the development of constitutional syphilis. Want or starvation, violent emotions, errors in diet, irritations of the intestinal mucous membrane by artificial articles of food or drink, abuse of spirits, excessive eating, want of exercise in the open air, fatiguing labor, forced marches, war, bivouacking, etc., excite the syphilitic dyscrasia.

On the contrary, the constitutional disease can be put off for a long time by rest, warmth, good clothes, suitable diet. These circumstances likewise favor the cure of the constitutional malady.

Although constitutional syphilis occurs more frequently among women than among men, yet it runs a more rapid course among the former. Pregnancy has a peculiar effect upon syphilis. During pregnancy, and particularly during the second period, new forms of the disease scarcely ever make their appearance. Existing forms of the disease either disappear of themselves or readily yield to treatment. Even when left to nature, they do not get worse until after parturition. This is particularly applicable as regards affections of the mucous membranes, skin, bones, glands, etc. Vegetations at the anus or sexual parts generally disappear of themselves towards the end of pregnancy, but exercise a so much more pernicious influence upon the fetus.

The signs of constitutional syphilis have a peculiar character, and on this account, are justly considered a *specific malady.* For instance, it is characteristic of this disease, only to affect certain organs, and even parts of organs, principally the mucous membrane of the mouth, fauces, nose, rectum and sexual organs; the skin and its appendages, the sub-cutaneous cellular tissue; the lymphatic system; the muscles and tendons; the brain and its membranes; the periosteum and the bones; the iris; the testicles and ovaries; the liver.

The constitutional disease is moreover distinguished by its form and color. The eruptions are generally of a *copper color, rounded,* disposed to form arched groups, or simple arches, rings, or serpentine lines, and giving rise to exudations which dry up and form crusts. Another peculiarity of the disease is, rarely to affect only one organ or tissue, but several tissues at the same time.

The skin and mucous membranes, and the lymphatic glands, are the most frequent seats of the constitutional disease in all its various forms, degrees and stages.

The development of the constitutional symptoms takes place in two successive periods, termed by Ricord *secondary* and *tertiary syphilis.*

Although these two forms of the constitutional syphilis are not separated by any distinct lines of demarcation, yet this distinction seems to be very convenient, and is very generally recognized by physicians. These two forms sometimes co-exist at one and the same period.

Secondary Syphilis.

In some cases, the first signs of constitutional syphilis appear during the existence of the primary chancre, especially the Hunterian or indurated form; generally, however, they break out a few months, and in a few rare cases, several years after the primary disease.

Careful observation would probably show that the first absorption of the poison by the general organism is accompanied by a feverish reaction, termed *syphilitic eruptive fever.* Afterwards it assumes all sorts of syphilitic inflammations and ulcerations, growths, indurations, etc. The mucous membranes are first invaded by these derangements, particularly the mucous membrane of the mouth, fauces, and the adjoining parts; afterwards the mucous membranes of the labia pudendi and vaginæ, or the outer skin in the shape of eruptions, termed *syphilides;* and finally the eye, especially the iris, causing *iritis syphilitica.*

The first development of constitutional syphilis is frequently announced by paleness of the patient, swelling of the lymphatic glands, especially on the neck, shifting pains of an apparently rheumatic or neuralgic character, various cutaneous eruptions peculiar to syphilis, falling off of the hair, iritis and febrile motions.

This peculiar eruptive fever, generally precedes with more or less distinctness, the appearance of constitutional affections of the skin and mucous membranes. The first sign of a general infection of the organism is a feeling of malaise throughout the body. Afterwards, a very violent headache is experienced, in the forehead, occiput, and sometimes over the whole head. The patient complains of an aching, burning, stinging pain, or a pain as if the head were pressed together with an iron band, or split in two. The pain becomes more and more intolerable, and a variety of other symptoms supervenes, such as heaviness and tearing in the shoulders, forearms, small of the back, legs and knees, excessive languor, restlessness, sleeplessness, coated tongue, thirst, constipation, hot skin which is constantly covered with a little moisture, quick and rapid pulse; the urine deposits a sediment. The cervical glands commence to swell. The cicatrices of the primary ulcers become darker, sensitive, they swell and grow larger and harder. In bed the pains either diminish or disappear altogether, particularly after the appearance of the constitutional symptoms. Recently Sigmund observed that the first appearance of the eruptive fever is frequently attended with symptoms of jaundice, which seem to be referable to the ulterior development of the liver affection.

I. Syphilitic diseases of the Mucous Membranes.

These diseases either appear in the form of *erythema* and *erosions* of the mucous membrane of the mouth, fauces, nasal cavity and sexual organs, or in the shape of *little blotches*, *flat tubercles* (mucous tubercles) of these membranes, or finally, as *deep-seated tubercles* and *ulcerous excavations* of the same.

Syphilitic Erythemata and Erosions of the Mucous Membranes.

These eruptions occur most frequently on the mucous membrane of the mouth and fauces. They constitute isolated, circumscribed, dark-red or copper-colored, not very elevated, inflamed spots or streaks on the mucous membrane, especially on that of the soft palate, tonsils, uvula, pharynx and larynx. The buccal cavity and the fauces become hot, a difficulty of swallowing and a burning sensation in the fauces; hoarseness and pain when talking are experienced, the patient coughs and hawks, the voice becomes snuffling or jarring, the mouth and throat feel dry. The inner surface of the lips and cheeks, the palate, tonsils, uvula, the posterior surface of the pharynx, look bluish-red, the follicles are swollen and engorged with blood. In the centre of the intensely-red spots we discover smaller insulated spots of a grayish-white color, which, upon close examination, are found to be erosions.

Similar derangements are perceived on the mucous membrane of the nasal cavity and of the sexual organs. The nose seems at first affected as in common catarrh, but the symptoms are really precursors of mucous tubercles, or the so called *plaques muqueuses.* On the internal layer of the prepuce, in the furrow behind the glans and round the meatus urinarius, these tubercles generally form small rounded erosions upon a bright copper-colored base, and flat margins gradually disappearing in the surrounding membrane, and secreting a grayish, purulent, fetid fluid. Similar phenomena are seen on the mucous membranes of the pudendum. In both sexes these erosions give rise to the formation of condylomata. At the anus, rhagades with a lardaceous bottom frequently develope themselves.

Among the remedies which are particularly adapted to this form of the syphilitic disease, the following are to be noticed: *Aconite,* (also during the eruptive fever,) *Anacardium, Arsen., Bellad., Aurum mur., Bryon., Calcarea carbon., Cannab., Canthar., Copaiv., Crot., Mercur. sol., Mercur. corros., Natrum carbon., Nitri. acid, Nux vom., Pulsat., Sulphur, Thuja.* Recently I have used *Anthrakokali* with advantage.

[*Acidum nitricum* is an excellent medicine in this affection, especially if the spots are dark-colored and disposed to bleed.

Mercurius sol. and corros., more particularly if no mercurial preparations had as yet been employed.

Aurum mur., if the syphilitic disease is complicated with symptoms of mercurial poisoning, in which case,

Sulphur may likewise prove serviceable, also *Hepar sulphuris.*

Arsenic will help, if gangrenous symptoms set in, or bad-looking scurfs cover the spots.

Kali hydriodicum is a most useful agent if the eruption shows a tendency to ulceration.]

Mucous Tubercles, Plaques Muqueuses.

These occur most frequently in females and children; in men they are less frequently noticed on the sexual organs and at the anus; in both sexes they develope themselves most frequently on the mucous membranes of the mouth and fauces. These mucous tubercles being still possessed of contagious properties and capable of developing by their secretion chancrous ulcers, they were for a long time looked upon as symptoms of primary syphilis.

They consist in flat, circumscribed elevations of the mucous membrane, which, together with its follicles and the submucous cellular tissue, is engorged and thickened, and secretes a tenacious, purulent exudation of a peculiar and extremely offensive odor. Their size varies from that of a millet-seed to the size of a dime. Sometimes several of them unite, forming irregularly-shaped, vaulted flakes. The smaller ones have altogether a tuberculoid shape, are generally very humid, regularly rounded, forming truncated cones, of a brighter redness in the centre than at the margin, and frequently are united in groups or regularly-shaped rings, especially on the glans, the inner surface of the cheeks and lips, the curtain of the palate, tongue, and at the roof of the mouth. The surrounding parts have a bluish-red, or bright copper-color.

The large tubercles are raised about a line above the mucous membrane, and either constitute perfectly round or more or less regularly oval, full, tense, and, on their upper surface, flattened elevations of the mucous membrane. Their color is a bright-red. On their surface they are covered with a thick, grayish-white layer of epithelium.

As we stated above, the mucous tubercles are rarely seen on the sexual organs of the male, and generally only singly or in ring-shaped groups. They appear much more frequently on the female parts, the labia majora and minora, at the entrance of the vagina, on the upper portion of the interior vagina, and even on the vaginal portion of the uterus. At the outer pudendum they occur either isolatedly or in crowds. Flat tubercles are likewise seen very frequently at the anus, even in children who had been abused for nefarious purposes.

The most destructive action of these tubercles takes place in the Schneiderian membrane. On account of the itching which they cause in this part, the crusts are scratched off, which gives rise to more obstinate ulcerations than in any other part. In many cases a portion of the wings of the nose is destroyed, which leaves a rugged surface and the Schneiderian membrane exposed.

If mucous tubercles develope themselves in the interior of the nose, the first symptoms are those of a catarrh which, however, last much longer than usual. A tickling and burning in the nose are experienced, and a watery fluid is secreted in great quantity; gradually a sensation supervenes as though it were difficult for the air to pass through the nose. The patients fancy the nose is full of mucus, and they blow it quite frequently. The whole mucous membrane becomes red, the faculty of smell is either diminished or arrested. Soon the tubercles ulcerate and become covered with a hard crust of irregular shape, varied thickness, reddish-brown color, and consisting of dried nasal mucus, blood and disorganized exudations. If proper means are not speedily and vigorously brought to bear upon this affection, the ulcers increase in size, grow larger and deeper, destroy the mucous membrane and the subjacent cellular tissue, perforate the septum and cause caries or necrosis of the nasal bones, cartilages, cribriform plate, etc. A quantity of fetid, greenish, bloody pus is discharged from the nose, (ozæna syphilitica;) the cartilages, upper jaw, vomer and the inner parts of the nose become invaded, disorganised, the hard palate is perforated, the nose disfigured, the speech becomes indistinct. The destructive process which is going on in these spongy bones, may extend to other parts of the head and vertebræ, and life may become endangered.

The following remedies have been found particularly useful for this affection:—

Acid nitricum, *Argent. nitr.*, *Bryon.*, *Calcar.*, *Ignat.*, *Pulsat.*, *Rhus tox.*, *Thuja.* If the tubercles are seated in the nose, the following medicines will be found most efficacious:—

Acidum nitr., *Acid. phosphor.*, *Argent. nitr.*, *Calcar. carb.*, *Kali carb.*, *Kreasot.*, *Lycop.*, *Mercur. corros.*, *Pulsat.*, *Rhus-tox.*, *Sepia*, *Staphys.*, *Sassapar.*, *Thuja.*

[Among these remedies the most important are undoubtedly the *mercurial preparations*, and if mercury had been used previously, and the symptoms are complicated with symptoms of mercurial poisoning, we may resort to *Acidum nitricum*, *Aurum muriaticum*, *Kali hydriodicum* and *Sepia*, in the order in which these remedies are here mentioned.]

Deep-seated tubercles and ulcerous excavations of the mucous membranes.

These ulcerations are almost always preceded by a tuberculous thickening of the mucous membrane and the submucous cellular tissue. The ulcers always penetrate to a considerable depth, destroy the mucous membrane throughout with great rapidity, and sometimes invade even the subjacent tissues. The ulcers are either isolated or in groups, rounded, and have sharply circumscribed, unequal, vaulted, pad shaped, and sometimes undermined margins. The bottom of the ulcers is frequently dotted with granulations, and like the margins, covered with a grayish or yellow, creamy, papescent, thick exudation.

These ulcerations occur principally in the neighborhood of the frænulum and on both sides of the glans. They may perforate the lower wall of the urethra, causing urinary fistulæ and strictures. At the female pudendum they are generally seated at the entrance of the vagina, the lower commissure, in the rugæ of the vagina, and on the vaginal portion of the uterus. On these parts they are apt to form abscesses which, if neglected, perforate the whole thickness of the vagina, spreading to the rectum and urethra, and causing recto-vaginal or urethro-vaginal fistulæ.

These ulcers occur moreover on the gums, in the nose, on

the tonsils, at the curtain of the palate, on the posterior wall of the fauces, at the epiglottis and in the larynx, causing more or less extensive disorganizations in these parts, and frequently terminating fatally.

The remedies which have been mentioned above for other forms of secondary syphilis, will, especially at the commencement, be found useful in this disease, if chosen with reference to the symptoms.

If the destructive process should have invaded the fauces and larynx, we may add the following remedies to the above mentioned list:—*Arsenic.*, *Carbo veg.*, *Natrum mur.*, and *Zinc. oxyd.*

II. Syphilitic exanthems, Syphilides, Exanthemata syphilitica.

The skin being a favorite seat of constitutional syphilis, it is not to be wondered that it should develope upon this organ a series of diversified morbid processes and eruptions which, for convenience of treatment, require to be distinguished into particular classes. We shall adopt the classification of the distinguished dermatologist Hebra, which, resting upon a pathologico-anatomical basis, is on this account to be considered the most expedient and useful.

Syphilitic eruptions have the general features of all other exanthems, but they occur principally in the shape of spots, pimples, tubercles, and fig warts. Sometimes they bear a striking resemblance to particular eruptions, such as measles, rubeolæ, varicellæ, lichen, psoriasis, variola, etc. In this case they may be distinguished by the following signs from similar non-syphilitic diseases: The syphilides run a characteristically slow but uninterrupted course which nothing can arrest. In most cases they come out in a definite number of efflorescences, and this number remains unchanged in their ulterior developments. Subsequent efflorescences appear at the same places where the former ones had dried up. Syphiloid eruptions are liable to relapses, but they always reappear at the same places. Their color is brown-red, resembling the color of copper or raw ham. Professor Hebra does not look upon this brown color as a characteristic sign of syphiloid eruptions. According to his opinion, this brown color arises from the frequent recurrence of these efflorescences at the same places and the depositions of pigment which always accompany the eruptions. From a similar cause, other non-syphilitic eruptions might exhibit a similar color, and this is indeed the case. The color of syphilides need not always be brown-red; if the pigment is yellow, the color of the eruption may be a mixture of yellow and red. It is a certain fact, however, that the color of syphiloid eruptions is always characterised by a sickly or dubious appearance, a sort of morbid discoloration. The color alone would not be a safe guide of diagnosis, but in conjunction with the other signs, it becomes an important symptom.

In regard to form, syphiloid eruptions prefer a circular shape. In the case of ulcerated eruptions of this class, the circular form is truly characteristic; first, they are kidney-shaped, and gradually assume a semi-lunar, and finally a semi-circular form.

Another peculiarity of syphilitic cutaneous diseases is this, that they form crusts in preference to scales. Such scales are generally thinner and drier than in non-syphilitic diseases. The crusts, on the contrary, are generally thick, large and deeply penetrating, and closely adhering to the subjacent parts. New crusts continuing to be added from day to day to the former layer, they gradually acquire an extraordinary thickness as in rupia. Syphiloid eruptions prefer such parts of the skin as are without adipose tissue, such as the head, forehead, (corona venerea,) occiput, nose, tibia; as a general rule they develope themselves on parts where other non-syphilitic eruptions are scarcely ever noticed. They become visible in the cold, and disappear during the warmth, particularly the roseola syphilitica. This is the contrary with non-syphilitic eruptions, which generally come out in warmth and disappear in the cold. Syphiloid eruptions do not itch; this is another of their peculiar characteristics, and reveals the syphilitic character of many eruptions which might otherwise pass for non-syphilitic. These eruptions constitute the first series of secundary syphilitic symptoms, and are sometimes accompanied by ulceration of the tonsils and pharyngeal mucous membrane, and in a few cases by bone-pains. Afterwards ulcerations of the laryngeal and nasal mucous membranes supervene.

As regards the classification of syphilides, the former method of arranging them under distinct heads with reference to their original or typical forms, is exceedingly inconvenient and impracticable; for these forms generally run into one another, and it frequently happens that several of them co-exist.

Hebra views the various forms of syphilides as certain stages of the syphilitic disease upon the skin; generally it first appears in the shape of spots; afterwards it assumes the tuberculoïd, then the squamous, fymatous, and other forms. According to Hebra, there are four or five positive periods during which the various forms of the syphiloid cutaneous disease gradually develope themselves.

Consequently we divide syphilides into

Erythemata (maculæ, syphilis cutanea maculosa;
Syphilis cutanea nodosa;
Syphilis cutanea squamosa, psoriasis;
Syph. cutan. papulosa;
Syphil. pustulosa, vesicles, blisters pustules;
Rupia syphilitica, crusts;
Condylomata;
Syphilitic affections of the hair and nails;

Maculæ, spots, ephelides.

This form is the most frequent and comes out first. The spots are separate, bright red, sometimes, however, they are very pale and only come out in the cold. Sometimes they are raised like blotches. Most ordinarily they appear on the chest, neck, face, arms, and in some cases on the inner side of the thighs, and in the neighborhood of the sexual organs;

other parts of the body are likewise liable to becoming the seats of these spots.

Not unfrequently they are accompanied by difficulty of swallowing, burning and dryness of the throat. They are distinguished from non-syphilitic spots, such as measles or rubeolæ, by this, that these non-syphilitic eruptions never become chronic, and generally disappear again after a period of from four to eight days. If the eruptions last longer, we may safely look upon them as syphilitic, roseola syphilitica.

This eruption runs a slow course, it is true, but never of five or six months; for previous to this it takes the form of tuberculoid syphilis. At certain periods, after eating, for instance, the spots grow larger. After having stood for some time, they generally grow paler, and the red color usually assumes a dirty gray, or gray-red tint.

Syphilitic cutaneous tubercles, flat tubercles or condylomata.

These tubercles are either single and incoherent, or else they form circular lines, or finally, they appear in groups or clusters. Very frequently they appear in company with mucous tubercles, principally on the scrotum, penis, mons veneris, in the inguinal folds, on the perinæum, round the anus, on the inside of the thighs, on the nape ef the neck, in the axillæ, on the hairy scalp, in the face, round the mouth, on the wings of the nose, on the forehead, between the toes, and along the nails. As a general rule, they only come out in one or the other of these places, only in a very few cases over the whole body. I have only seen one case of this kind, at Professor Hebra's clinique for cutaneous diseases.

The secretion which is discharged by these tubercles, continues in most cases contagious, not only for others, but also for the adjoining portions of the skin and mucous membrane of the patient himself. Generally they are of a bright copper-red color, and almost always painless. They develope themselves slowly and remain unaltered for a long time. Not unfrequently an ulcer forms on the surface of the tubercle, which becomes covered with a hard crust that leaves a deep cicatrix after falling off. If the tubercles do not ulcerate, they usually become depressed and flat, and assume a scaly form.

Squamous syphilis, scales, psoriasis.

Generally, this form arises from the tuberculoid form, and sometimes from the spots. The tubercles pass into large, irregularly-shaped, and sometimes confluent elevations of a bright copper color; they are covered with hard, readily-tearing scales, of a dull white color. As the disease progresses, the eruption loses its bright color, and only the scales remain. This usually takes place in the face, in the hollow of the hand (psoriasis palmaris), and on the soles of the feet (psoriasis plantaris.) In the palm of the hand the patient first sees brown-red spots; after a while, while washing himself, the patient imagines he observes callous risings above these spots. These risings are scratched off by the patient; they come off in the shape of scales, after a while the livid spots and risings return, are scratched off a second time, after which rhagades and then ulcers form. Ulcers are very apt to arise from any form of syphilitic efflorescences.

Papulæ, lichen.

We distinguish large and small papulæ. The small papulæ constitute miliary, acuminated, hard elevations on the skin, which are disposed to pass into suppuration or to assume the form of acne syplilitica. These papulæ generally form round, circular or arched groups of a bright-red copper color, and frequently come out in innumerable quantity. The eruption of the papulæ is almost always preceded by fever. The exanthem may develope itself on every part of the body, but it appears most frequently on the extremities, back, nape of the neck, shoulders, on the parts adjoining the sexual parts, and on the lower surface of the penis, less frequently in the face and on the neck.

The large papulæ appear most frequently on the extremities, shoulders, nape of the neck, chest, forehead and hairy scalp; sometimes on all these parts at one and the same period. Generally it remains unaltered for several months. Unless arrested by proper treatment, the eruption keeps renewing itself constantly. Previous to the appearance of the papulæ, small, reddish-yellow spots of a regularly round shape appear upon the skin, either singly, scattered over a large space, or, more rarely in clusters. Upon these spots start up slowly and in a perpendicular direction, acuminated, hard, globular, lenticular callosities, from one to two lines in diameter, and of a bright copper color. Soon they reach the size of a pea, and are so closely crowded together that the place where they are located constitutes an elevation upon the skin. In some cases they constitute rings of various sizes raised above the skin, and generally of a rounded shape. The open sides of the adjoining rings are sometimes in opposite directions, so that, if the terminal points of the lines communicate, a serpentine or wave-line is formed. Sometimes the papulæ form scales, under which ulcers are seldom witnessed.

The large papulæ are frequently accompanied by ulcers in the fauces, inflammation of the iris, papulous eruptions on the mucous membranes of the sexual organs, especially the mucous membrane of the glans.

Syphilitic pustules, vesicles, blisters, bullæ.

Syphilitic vesicles are an extremely rare disease; among 1000 cases scarcely one occurs. Prof. Hebra who is at the head of one of the most extensive cliniques of Europe for cutaneous diseases, has never yet seen such a case. This impartial observer maintains that herpes is never of syphilitic origin; a syphilitic eczema would not cause any itching, and would gradually terminate in ulceration; but every eczema does cause an itching, hence it cannot be syphilitic. At all events the existence of this form is doubtful.

This remark does not apply to the other syphilides with liquid exudations, such as syphilitic pustules, bullæ, blisters, pemphigus, ecthyma and impetigo pustulo-crustacea.

Syphilitic pustules take the form of acne syphilitica in young, robust, plethoric persons, while the parts surrounding the pustules are of an intensely bright-red color, and the secretion of pus takes place more rapidly. The larger pustules, with a pit in the centre, marked by a small, black, drying-up point, can scarcely be distinguished from variola, and are on this account termed variola syphilitica. In children who were infected by their nurses, they came out in the face, on the abdomen and thighs, in the shape of a superficial ecthyma. They soon break in these cases, forming bright-yellow loosely adhering crusts. In old or young impoverished constitutions the pustules develope themselves very slowly, every single pustule being surrounded by a light blue-red, livid tint.

Syphilitic pustules are very apt to occur after other syphilides, such as papulæ or tubercles.

Syphilitic variola is distinguished from genuine variola by this, that the former keeps breaking out anew in successive intervals; that the crusts do not fall off at one and the same period, and that this process lasts longer than in common variola. Except this, the pustules have the same shape and size, and cover the same parts of the body, as the common variola. They break out and run their course without any fever. In some cases, however, the pustules are so large that they cannot be mistaken for small-pox.

Syphilitic varicella appears most frequently in the face, on the abdomen, on the inner side of the thighs, and on the legs, less frequently on the arms. This eruption is generally preceded by a violent fever, on which account it might readily be confounded with varicella. After the fever has lasted two or three days, spots break out on several parts of the body in succession; they are round, of a pale-red, seldom of a bright-copper color, and soon are raised above the skin throughout their whole extent, and, in their interior, contain a bright-yellow of whitish fluid. Afterwards a copper-colored circular areola forms around the pustules.

The syphilitic pemphigus is generally noticed in children,

less frequently in full-grown persons. It is composed of blisters of the size of beans, and of an irregular shape. These blisters generally break, leaving ulcers which, by the matter which continues to exude, and by a want of cleanliness, form crusts that frequently increase to an enormous size and constitute the rupia syphilitica. It is not necessarily the case, however, for every rupia to be preceded by pemphigus. The rupia may come on after any syphilitic ulcer. According to Hebra, the pemphigus of new-born infants is not necessarily syphilitic. He maintains that pemphigus is a disease sui generis, that it breaks out in other parts than those which are generally selected by the syphilitic disease, and that it attacks mostly small children who die from its effects. Successive breakings out do not take place in the case of pemphigus; in some cases ulcers appear after the blisters, in other cases they are wanting. The pemphigus of new-born infants always contains gaëlic acid according to Dr. Schottin; that of full-grown persons never contains any.

Pemphigus is generally seated on the sexual organs, on the abdomen and extremities, less frequently in the palms of the hands and on the soles of the feet. It breaks out in superficial, bloch-shaped risings of the skin, of a bright copper color; the blisters are surrounded by a copper-colored or violet areola, and always leave yellow, transparent crusts behind.

The next variety, *impetigo pustulo-crustacea*, is frequently seen accompanied with affections of the mucous membrane of the nose and mouth. The pustules are crowded together in large numbers, and run into one another. Thick, large crusts form, with ulcers underneath that secrete a tolerably large quantity of pus, and leave large scattered cicatrices. They mostly appear on the chest, neck, in the face, at the eyebrows and on the forehead. The pustules are preceded by a more or less bright redness; after a while small, rounded, purulent tips become visible in close proximity to each other and running into each other the more rapidly the more the skin is inflamed. The pustules which are filled with the purulent secretion, soon break, the discharged pus dries up to one or more greenish crusts of large size, thick, not much raised above the skin, surrounded by a copper-colored areola and yielding to the pressure of the finger.

The *ecthyma* is characterised by larger pustules than the former. The pustules are circular, conical, from three to four lines in diameter, and containing a thick, green-yellow pus. The areola which surrounds the pustules, is of a striking copper-color, but not very hard. The pustules soon break, and become covered with a brown, rounded, loosely-adhering crust of uniform thickness, under which a superficial ulcer is seated. The ecthyma is mostly found on the hairy scalp, on the parts round the mouth and on the forearms, but it may likewise break out on any other part of the body, and spread over a considerable extent of surface. If the ecthymatous pustules are very large, oval, they form a transition link with the next following eruption, rupia syphilitica.

Rupia Syphilitica.

The rupia frequently arises from pemphigus or ecthyma, but it may likewise break out without any of these forms preceding it. In the former case it arises from blisters of a regularly round shape, of the size of beans, not very tense, and surrounded by a copper-colored areola; they stand upon a swollen, indurated basis, and contain a dark-yellow, purulent fluid, which changes to a brownish color. The pus dries up in the middle of the blister, and forms a small brown crust. Round the crust the epidermis likewise rises in blisters filled with a similar brownish-red, purulent fluid; these likewise dry up, thus enlarging the crust in extent, whilst its enlargement in depth is promoted by the drying up of the recent exudations in the interior of the pustules; by this means the crust gradually acquires a conical or pyramidal shape. The crusts sometimes increase to an extraordinary size, but they are not very numerous; there are at most from twelve to twenty crusts scattered over the whole body. They run a very slow course, and, on account of the secretion of pus which is continually going on under the crusts, undermine the patient's constitution, so that, after a while, the patients grow so feeble, that they are scarcely able to walk, the digestive functions are impaired, and a supervening diarrhœa hastens the final dissolution of the patient.

The *serpiginous* and *perforating* tubercles are related to this form of syphilides. Either of the former eruptions is greatly disposed to destroy the tissue of the skin. Either commences with nodous swellings extending into the subcutaneous cellular tissue. The serpiginous tubercles are large, hard, and have a pretty regular, round shape. Perforating tubercles only exist in small number, forming spheroidal risings on the skin, and penetrating to the sub-cutaneous cellular tissue, where they can be felt with the finger as hard tumors.

Serpiginous tubercles occur most frequently in the face, on the nape of the neck, on the head, forehead, shoulders and trunk, less frequently on the rest of the body, but never on the borders or soles of the feet. By successive growth they may gradually spread over a large portion of the surface of a part or of one side of the trunk. Serpiginous tubercles have at first a bright copper-color and a shining surface, which is never covered with scales. Afterwards they become inflamed, ulcers form at their tips and become covered with a thick, hard, conical, brownish or yellowish-gray, firmly-adhering crust. If the crust is detached, we discover a superficial ulcer with a grayish bottom, which is speedily covered with a new, softer, and less dark-colored crust.

The *perforating tubercles* occur most frequently in scrofulous individuals with a delicate, white skin, generally in the face, on the cheeks, round the nose and lips, in front of the ear, on the legs, and also on other parts of the body.

Both these forms of tubercles are greatly disposed to passing into the form of ulcers; those arising from perforating tubercles frequently destroy the skin entirely.

In few cases the perforating tubercles appear on the nasal wings and lips in groups of several crowded together; this causes the surrounding parts to swell, and imparts to the ulcer the appearance of lupus or cancer, with which they are frequently confounded. These two eruptions are the most dilatory in breaking out after the primary syphilis; sometimes six, eight, ten and more years elapse before they make their appearance.

Condylomata syphilitica, papules muqueuses, (Ricord,) tubercules syphilitiques plates, (Rayer,) pustules plates, (Cullerier,) figwarts.

The original nature of condylomata is not yet settled to the satisfaction of all parties. Some consider them of syphilitic origin, whereas others maintain that they may exist without any syphilitic taint. This is likewise our opinion; we have seen a number of condylomata which were evidently non-syphilitic, inasmuch as not a trace of either primary or secondary syphilis was perceptible in the organism.

The condylomata are either raised and acuminated, or broad and flat; they always arise from morbidly enlarged papillæ of the corion, which are covered with a thickened epidermis.

We generally distinguish two kinds of figwarts, according as they are seated upon a broad or narrow basis. The *broad condylomata* are of syphilitic origin, the *acuminated* condylomata are non-syphilitic, and may be caused by the irritating action of coït, by want of cleanliness, gonorrhœa or leucorrhœa, they are generally more obstinate than those with a broad base. Some maintain that the broad condylomata are hypertrophied conditions of the skin, and that the acuminated condylomata are parasites.

Fricke and Hauck adopt another class of condylomata, the subcutaneous, consisting of condylomatous swellings in the mucous and cuticular follicles. Hauck says in this respect: "In young individuals with a delicate skin, especially in young females who had been affected with gonorrhœa, leucorrhœa, or with acuminated condylomata, but not merely with chancre, we frequently notice on the internal surface of the thighs down to the knees, on the outer skin of the penis and of the labia majora, on the mons veneris and on the abdomen, but no where else, *small, rather hard and elastic, yellowish-white elevations, of the size of a millet-seed, and about two lines in height, somewhat smaller at the upper extremity which is flat, and upon which a dark, dot-shaped depression is visible.* On account of their external appearance, these tubercles were termed by Fricke *syphilitic porcelain tubercles.*

Hauck discovered the real nature of the subcutaneous figwarts by the following experiment: Placing both thumb-nails against the base of the cutaneous elevation, he pressed them together from above downwards, upon which the thickened and whitish sebaceous contents started in vermicular shape out of the opened follicle. Upon renewing the pressure the small follicle was again opened, a small, whitish, globular, compressed, crisp, sometimes pluri-lobular growth, started out of the interior, which was at once recognized as an acuminated condyloma, adhering by its root to the bottom of the follicle, but being otherwise perfectly disconnected from the surrounding parts.

According to Barensprung, Simon, Kræmer and others, condylomata constitute a degeneration of single portions of the skin, particularly of the epidermis, the papillæ and the hairy follicles. Upon some circumscribed spot the papillæ first grow uniformly larger, and the epidermis covering this part grows thicker, so that the original condyloma constitutes a flat and smooth elevation upon the skin. On portions of the skin which are more remote from the mucous membranes, particularly on the scrotum, the condylomata seldom advance beyond this stage; but on parts which are nearer to the mucous membrane, the development of the condylomata takes place much more rapidly. Towards the end the elongated papilla forms bulbous swellings; these give out shoots, which in their turn give out other shoots, and in this way a papillæ which was simple at its base, is gradually transformed into a tissue of numerous ramifications. Every papillæ contains a blood vessel.

The more extensive these condylomata become, the thinner becomes the epidermis, which, however, never disappears entirely. In most cases the epidermis which is thoroughly pervaded by fluid, resembles the epithelium of the mucous membranes.

The *variety of the forms* depends upon the *shape and the extent of that portion of the skin which was originally diseased.* If this portion is small, *acuminated*, and if large, *broad* condylomata arise from it. At other times the variety of the forms depends upon the *manner in which* the ramifications shoot up, and upon the *locality*. If these ramifications shoot out longitudinally, in this case the condyloma takes the form of a cone, standing upon its pointed extremity; if they are developed in every direction indiscriminately, the condylomata assume the shape of raspberries; at the anus the condylomatous growths like to accommodate themselves to the natural folds of the skin, and being flattened on either side, they assume the shape of a cock's comb. If these growths spread over a large surface in every direction, they form *cauliflower-shaped*, *pedunculated*, *fig-shaped*, *mulberry-shaped*, *fungous*, *grape-shaped*, or other kinds of condylomatous excrescences.

Condylomata, whether syphilitic or non-syphilitic, most frequently attack persons who do not keep themselves clean, on parts of the skin or mucous membranes, where two flat surfaces from which corrosive secretions ooze out, come in contact with, or rub against each other. They occur more frequently on the female than on the male parts. We see them on the labia majora and minora, at the entrance of the vagina, in the vagina, in the rugæ of the vaginal mucous membrane, at the roof of the vagina, etc. There are cases where the whole vagina is dotted with such comdylomata. In the male sex we see them in the furrow behind the corona glandis, on the glans, in the meatus urinarius. Favorite localities of the condylomata, in both sexes, are the inner surface of the anus and the surrounding parts, and the perinæum; here too they are more frequently in females than in males. They are likewise observed in the corners of the mouth and lips, in the nose, mouth and fauces, in the external meatus auditorius, on the conjunctiva of the eye, upon the skin of the inner side of the thighs, in the inguinal folds, in the axilla, and even, though rarely, on the fingers.

Syphilitic affections of the hair and nails. Alopecia syphilitica and *onychia maligna syphilitica.*

General or partial falling off of the hair, especially on the head, with furfuraceous desquamation, occurs in various periods of constitutional syphilis, but most frequently as a consequence of syphiloid eruptions. At first the hair comes out more abundantly only when combing it; afterwards the hair not only comes out on the head, but also at the eyebrows, eyelashes, whiskers and the sexual parts. The skin on these parts is covered with thin, whitish or bright-yellow scales, which constantly form anew. The whole affected portion of the skin looks redder. The hair which grows out in the place of that which had fallen off, is thinner, of a lighter color, it remains small and frizzles. In young persons it acquires again its former consistence and rich growth as soon as the constitutional disease is healed. In old persons it remains thin and small as long as they live. The falling off of the hair is promoted by the use of mercury.

While the syphilitic diseases is running into the tertiary form, the onychia syphilitica is frequently added to the other symptoms. It is especially the nodous form of cutaneous syphilis that is disposed to invade the nails. The patients experience pains in the fingers, especially in the thumb; the least pressure is intolerable. Afterwards a small, semilunar ulcer forms with its convex surface turned upwards; the pain and sensitiveness become exceedingly acute, the ulcer enlarges in size, the whole root of the nail is affected and the nail is finally destroyed without ever growing again.

Onychia syphilitica invades the fingers as well as the toes, but principally the latter. In most cases several nails are diseased; it has happened that every nail of the upper and lower extremities was destroyed.

In conducting the treatment of any of these secundary eruptions of the syphilitic disease, the diet should be constantly in accordance with the strictest homœopathic treatment. What is of still more importance than the diet is this, that the patient should be kept in an uniform, somewhat elevated temperature. In the warmer climate of the South, syphiloid eruptions run a much more rapid and more favorable course, and the cure is much more readily accomplished than in the colder North.

Among the remedies which we shall mention for the syphilitic dyscrasia, one or more, in alternation or succession, will have to be prescribed in accordance with the symptoms. We have to remember that the syphilides are disposed to pass from one into another, and that several forms frequently coexist. The proper mode of alternating the drugs, their succession or the repetition of the dose, will have to be left to the discretion of the practitioner or the intelligent layman.

In erythema, roseola syphilitica, the following remedies will be found most suitable: ANTIM. CRUD., *Arnic.*, *Arsen.*, *Aurum*, *Bellad.*, *Calc. carb.*, CANTHARIS., *Chelid.*, *Chin. sulph.*, *Clemat.*, *Coccul.*, COPAIV., *Crot. tigl.*, *Lycop.*, MERC. SOL., MERC. CORROS., *Mezereum*, *Petrol.*, *Phosphor.*, TART. EMET.

In nodous syphilis, flat condylomata, we may use: *Antim. crud.*, AURUM, *Bovista*, *Carbo anim.*, *Carbo veget.*, *Caustic.*, *Hepar sulph.*, *Kali carb.*, *Ledum*, MER. SOL., *Nitr.*, STAPHY., *Thuja.*

For psoriasis syphilitica we recommend: *Baryt. mur.*, *Copaiva*, *Cuprum*, *Calc. carb.*, *Calc. acet.*, HEPAR SULPH., *Kali carb.*, *Mezer.*, MERCUR., *Natr. carb.* NITR. ACID., *Plumbum*, *Graph.*, *Gratiola.* (Also, KALI HYDRIODICUM.)

In papulous syphilis we use with advantage: *Agaric*, *Ammon. mur.*, *Arsen.*, *Aurum*, *Bovist*, *Caustic.*, *Con.*, COPAIV., *Graphit.*, *Iod.*, *Kali. carb.*, KALI HYDRIOD., *Ledum.*, *Lycop.*,

MERC., *Nat. carb.*, *Nat. mur.*, *Phosphor.*, *Rhus. tox.*, *Stramon.*, *Tabac.*, *Tereb.*, ZINCUM.

In pustulous syphilis, variola syphilitica, ecthyma syphiliticum, we have: *Acid. nitr.*, ANTIM. CRUD., *Amm. mur.*, *Argent. nitr.*, *Arsen.*, *Bellad.*, *Baryt. carb.*, *Bryon.*, *Caustic.*, *Calc. carb.*, CANTHAR., *Carbo. veg.*, *Clemat.*, *Coccul.*, *Copaiv.*, *Crot.*, *Dros.*, *Evonyn.*, *Graph.*, *Hyos.*, *Kali hydriod.*, *Kali carb.*, MERC. SOL., MERC. CORROSIVUS, *Mezer.*, *Natr. mur.*, *Phosphor.*, *Petrol.*, *Ranunc. bulb.*, *Ranunc. sceler.*, *Rhus. tox.*, SASSAPAR., *Secale corn.*, *Tabac.*, *Tereb.*

For rupia syphilitica the following seven remedies have been found efficacious: ACID. MUR., *Arsen.*, *Caustic.*, *Crot.*, DULCAM., *Rhus tox.*, *Sabina.*

Condylomata are controlled with tolerable certainty by *Aurum*, *Causticum*, *Phosphoric acid*, MERC. SOL., THUJA., and SABINA.

Alopecia syphilitica requires: *Arsen.*, *Calc. carb.*, *Carbo. veg.*, *Graph.*, *Hyper.*, *Iod.*, *Kali carb.*, LYCOP., *Magnesia carb.*, MERCUR., *Natr. mur.*, NITRI ACID., *Petrol.*, *Phosphor.*, *Selen.*, *Sepia*, *Sulphur.*

To onychia syphilitica the following remedies are adapted: *Arsen.*, *Antim. crud.*, GRAPHIT., *Hep. sulph.*, *Kali carb.*, *Lycop.*, MERC., SOL., *Nux vom.*, *Petrol.*

(Among the above named remedies those which are printed in fat type, have the nearest resemblance to the disease, and may, as a general rule, be tried first. In all syphilitic diseases the Mercurial preparations occupy the first rank. Acidum nitricum and Iodine, with their compounds, are likewise powerful anti-syphilitica, and deserve especial attention in the case of mercurial complications; this remark likewise applies to Aurum and its compounds. Next to these we have Silicea, Mezereum, Acidum phosphoricum, and the class of remedies generally indicated for scrofulosis and tuberculosis.)

III. IRITIS SYPHILITICA.

This disease is intermediate between secondary and tertiary syphilis, and is by some authors reckoned among the former, by others among the latter variety. Ricord places it among the forms of secundary syphilis. We feel disposed to do the same, for we have often met it in conjunction with roseola, lichen and other syphilides. According to Helbert, about four out of every hundred patients affected with secundary syphilis are attacked with iritis. There are, however, syphilitic eye-diseases, and iritis is one them, which are evidently forms of tertiary syphilis. These diseases will be treated of in detail in the chapter on tertiary syphilis.

We will now go into some details regarding secundary iritis.

This disease is characterized by a very violent inflammation of the membrane of Descemet, especially on the anterior surface of the iris, which results in dimness of the cornea, yellowish or greenish discoloration of the iris, contraction or distortion of the pupil, morbid dilatation thereof (mydriasis), excessive photophobia and nocturnal pains in the orbit.

In most cases syphilitic iritis affects one eye only, and has all the properties and appearances of common iritis.

In the commencement of the disease, the color of the iris becomes duller, grayish, the smaller circle is less clearly distinguished from the larger, the radii are more or less effaced. The pupil is moved with difficulty, more or less contracted, its shape is altered, angular. The cornea is somewhat dimmed and on the inner surface we discover a few bundles of vessels.

The whole of the sclerotica is filled with blood, of a rose color; at its juncture with the cornea we perceive a dark-red, more or less broad, violently inflamed, ring. The patients complain of a drawing and a dull pressure in the eye, photophobia, increased secretion of tears; the sight is blurred as if a gauze were before the eyes,

After a while these changes become more intense and spread. The iris becomes more discolored, almost of a dirty-red color. This change is particularly distinct in the case of gray and blue eyes; blue eyes generally change to a greenish-red. The surface of the iris is lined by a layer of exudation of more or less thickness; this causes the iris to swell, its free margin is thickened, and upon its anterior surface we discover globular elevations of a yellow or gray color. The pupil is perfectly immovable, contracted and distorted. In the substance of the iris we discover small extravasations of blood, abscesses, forming upon its anterior surface small, rounded, yellow elevations, and at its free margin reddish-yellow, roundish flocks or globular, pedunculated excrescenses, termed *condylomata of the iris.* As the disease progresses, adhesions take place between the iris and the lenticular capsule. If, in such a case, the pupil still remains open, it does not look black but grayish. At the bottom of the anterior chamber we observe through the dim cornea a more or less elevated layer of pus which is sometimes mixed with blood. As the disorganization progresses, the pain increases in violence. The patient experiences violent, constrictive, boring pains and stitches spreading to the temples, forehead and even the cheeks. The pains are worse in the evening and at night, so that the patients have scarcely ever any sleep. If the disease is not speedily arrested, it may spread to the other membranes of the eye, causing amaurosis, specks on the cornea, stamphyloma, mydriasis, etc. The lighter degrees of iritis are speedily controlled by judicious treatment; but there remains a tendency to relapses, on which account the patients have to observe great caution for some time to come.

In treating the disease, we have above all things to protect the eye from the light. This is done by wearing a green screen before the eye, and by abstaining from any work that might strain the eye, such as reading or writing. It may even be necessary to keep the patient constantly in a dark room.

Among the homœopathic remedies the principal is *Merc. sol.*, provided the patient had not been drugged with mercury by some allopathic physician. If this should have been the case, we have to give: *Acid. nitr.*, *Aurum*, *Belladonna*, *Cannabis*, *Carbo veg.*, *Crocus*, *Coffea*, *Graphit.*, *Hepar sulph.*, *Kali carb.*, *Lycop.*, *Pulsat.*, *Sulph.*, *Thuja*, *Veratr.*

[It is doubtful whether such agents as Crocus and Coffea will be of any direct use in syphilitic iritis; the remedies from which positive benefit may be derived in this affection, are *Acidum nitricum*, *Mercurius solubilis* and *corrosivus*, and, if there should be intense pain in the frontal region, and rapid distortion of the pupil, the saturated tincture of the root of Aconite. It is well to use this agent in alternation with Mercurius corrosivus.]

Tertiary Syphilis.

According to Ricord, the symptoms of tertiary syphilis differ from those of secundary syphilis in this, that they are no longer transmissible to the fetus. Ricord maintains that, at this period, the syphilitic disease loses its specific character, and that it becomes a dyscrasia which is very much analogous to scrofulosis. The older the syphilis, and the longer it lasts, the more it becomes divested of its specific character. Tertiary symptoms are always preceded by primary and secondary phenomena. Physicians who dispute this point, have certainly forgotten to institute a careful subjective and objective analysis.

Tertiary symptoms are much more formidable than the conditions by which they were preceded, and are the more serious the longer and more diversified had been the anti-syphilitic cures which the patients had undergone. The mercurial treatment, especially, renders the tertiary symptoms inveterate. Mercury enfeebles the body, and the syphilitic disease is the more frightful the more debilitated the constitution in which it exercises its ravages.

Tertiary symptoms seldom show themselves under six months after the disappearance of the chancre. This is the shortest period. As to the period beyond which the action of the syphilitic poison need no longer be apprehended, it is impossible to determine it with any thing like certainty. Cases have occurred where the syphilitic disease broke out ten, fifteen, twenty years after the first infection; but such a long period rarely ever elapses without the occasional supervention of suspicious symptoms. There is always some little trouble which the patient overlooks on account of its insignificance. But suddenly the disease breaks out; a steady pain is felt in one of the tibiæ, or a testicle begins to swell.

Tertiary symptoms affect the sub-cutaneous and sub-mucous cellular tissue, the fibrous, osseous and cartilaginous tissues, the muscles, nerves, parenchymatous organs; in short, the whole organism.

Accordingly, we distinguish affections of the sub-cutaneous and sub-mucous tissue, of the cellular tissue, and of the lymphatic glands and vessels enclosed in it.

Tertiary symptoms of the fibrous and parenchymatous organs.

Syphilitic diseases of the periosteum and bones.

Syphilitic affections of the muscles and tendons.

Syphilitic affections of the eyes.

Syphilitic affections of the nerves.

Syphilitic affections of parenchymatous organs and syphilitic cachexia.

I. Tertiary Affections of the Sub-cutaneous and Sub-mucous Tissue, the Cellular Tissue, the Lymphatic Glands and Vessels.

Gummata Syphilitica, Gummatose Tumors on the Skin and in Parenchymatous Organs.

These tumors are located in the sub-cutaneous, sub-mucous or interstitial cellular tissue. They are found more frequently under the skin or under the mucous membranes than more deep-seated. They are not often met with, belong to the remotest stage or period of constitutional syphilis, and not unfrequently accompany syphilitic cachexia. They run a slow course, and are liable to relapses.

Gummata occur most frequently under the scalp, the skin of the neck, upper arms, legs, especially on the inside of the thighs and legs, on the prepuce and under the skin of the penis and scrotum. At first we observe a pea-shaped, round, very hard, not very prominent swelling under the skin; whose color is not altered in the least. These swellings are painless, and it is only during a change of weather that a slight, dull pain is experienced in the part where they are seated. They increase slowly in size; sometimes a year elapses before they reach the size of a hazel-nut. They seldom occur singly, but are generally disposed in a row, like beads, from four to six together. For a long time they remain hard, can be moved to and fro over the subjacent parts, but their upper surface firmly adheres to the skin. These swellings frequently remain unaltered for years. Finally, however, in one case sooner, in the other later, they become soft. In the centre of the tumor pus begins to form, and this change keeps spreading to the circumference. In the meanwhile the gumma has formed adhesions with the adjoining parts, and is enclosed as in a kind of cyst. The process of softening takes place in the interior of the cyst, and, after awhile, fluctuation is perceived through the walls of the cyst, and becomes more and more distinct. Gradually the formerly hard gumma acquires the consistence of an abscess filled with pus. The skin over the swelling, the color of which had remained unaltered so far, now changes to a bluish copper-color, becomes thinner, breaks, and a fetid ichor is discharged from the tumor. This ichorous exudation sometimes undermines the neighboring cellular tissue, forming widely-ramified fistulous canals. At this period, the discharge of ichor is generally accompanied with portions of organized tissue. The ulcerative process extends more and more, both in breadth and depth, the edges of the ulcer look suspicious.

Gummata of the sub-mucous cellular tissue of the tongue deserve especial mention. Syphilitic tumors of the tongue are frequently confounded with diseases of an entirely different nature. They have been mistaken for cancer and schirrus, and have been cut out. These sub-mucous gummata of the tongue develope themselves without the patient being made aware of it by any symptom of pain. The tongue becomes hard, knotty, either in one portion only or throughout its whole extent. The free motion of the tongue in talking or chewing is of course impeded. These swellings may be distinguished from cancer by the absence of the shooting pains which are always felt in the latter.

The most suitable remedy for these gummata is undoubtedly *Merc. sol.* which will always have the desired effect, provided the patient had not been drugged with allopathic doses of calomel. If this remedy should not suffice, one or more of the following remedies will have to be chosen: *Arsenic, Borax, China, Mezer., Mecur. dulc., Plumb., Stramon., Rhus tox., Ruta, Carbo anim., Aurum, Belladonna, Acidum phosphor., Calcar. carbon., Graphit., Juglans.*

Symptomatic Indications.

[*Arsenicum* is particularly indicated when the suppurative process has already commenced, and symptoms of a malignant character are developed; the pus is ichorous, thin, corrosive, foul, and the swelling has a livid appearance.

China may be used after arsenic, if this should not help, or in alternation with it; and if neither arsenic nor china should make any impression, and the character of the pus should remain unchanged, or if the tumor should seem to be perfectly torpid and hard,

Carbo animalis may be employed with great advantage.

Mercurius dulcis may be given after Mercurius sol. had been tried ineffectually.

Rhus tox. is excellent when the swelling is hard as stone, or when a commencement of torpid inflammation becomes visible.

Aurum may be tried after Mercury, in case this agent should not have any effect, or in case mercury should have been given previously, or by some allopathic practitioner. In such a case

Nitri acidum, Calcarea carbonica, Acidum phosphoricum and *Graphites* might likewise be given with advantage. These remedies are likewise useful if the swelling does not seem to be impressed in the least by any of the previously named remedies.]

Belladonna is indicated when the swelling looks inflamed, and is very tender and hot, or a throbbing is experienced in the tumor.

Juglans is indicated when the swelling begins to feel sore, or symptoms of ulceration develope themselves. In such a case

Mezereum, *Calcarea carb.*, and *Graphites* will likewise prove useful.]

II. Tertiary Affections of the Fibrous and Parenchymatous organs.

Sarcocele syphilitica, orchitis syphilitica, syphilitic swelling of the testes.

For a long time syphilitic sarcocele was looked upon as identical with orchitis arising from gonorrhœa. The difference between these two forms of orchitis was first scientifically and thoroughly accounted for by Astley Cooper, Dupuytren, but particularly by Ricord. In speaking of this disease we shall adopt the masterly description by Ricord, which is distinguished by clearness and correctness; without, however, neglecting the more recent observations and views of Hamilton, Helot and Moore.

According to Ricord syphilitic sarcocele which has also been termed albuginea syphilitica, because the tunica albuginea is principally affected in this disease, constitutes one of the first and most frequent symptoms of tertiary syphilis. It usually affects one side only, although cases occur where both testicles, or one after the other, are diseased. There are scarcely ever any precursory symptoms; now and then, but in a few cases only, the patients complain of acute boring pains in the loins, generally at night; sometimes they complain of a painful pressure in the region of the kidneys, or of a sensation as if a sticking instrument were thrust through their flesh. In some cases the nocturnal appearance of the pains denotes an evidently syphilitic origin. As a general rule, however, the precursory symptoms are wanting; the testicle begins to swell without the patient being at all aware of it. Some, however, have their attention called to the approaching trouble by a sensation of troublesome tension and a dull pain in the testicles prior to any appearance of swelling. Most frequently the alteration is unaccompanied by any striking phenomena, and developes itself in the following manner: in the testicle which is the seat of the disease, we discover one or more indurated nodes; on pressing the testicle we feel a small spot that is harder and less elastic than the other parts. As the disease progresses, this induration continues to spread. In many cases the induration spreads round about like a circular belt; in other cases several indurations make their appearance successively and gradually coalesce until the whole testicle has become involved.

In simple cases, where the sarcocele runs a regular course, the epididymis remains unaltered for a long period, and can be clearly distinguished from the testicle proper which either preserves its normal volume while the induration is going forwards, or becomes hypertrophied. But even if the testicle swells, the swelling never goes beyond certain limits, and this is another diagnostic sign of syphilitic sarcocele, for in many other forms of disorganization of the testes, such as elephantiasis, fungous enlargement, this organ may acquire an enormous size.

The increase of the swelling in syphilitic sarcocele takes place with great regularity. The testicle preserves its pear-shaped form, the larger extremity being turned downwards, and the elongated extremity upwards, and the longitudinal diameter in the direction of the spermatic cord. The syphilitic testicle feels harder than the other; the hypertrophy is regular; the inequalities which we discover with the finger, observe a certain regularity; they constitute a regularly progressive series of circular or zone-shaped indurations. As soon as the swelling has reached three or four times the size of the original testicle, the epididymis is no longer perceptible even upon close examination; an oval swelling is all that we discover; nevertheless the epididymis is not morbidly altered; neither the epididymis nor the vas deferens is involved in any degree in the process of degeneration.

This is a very important diagnostic sign; for degeneration of the epididymis or spermatic cord would constitute a most unusual complication. If the sarcocele attains a certain degree, the testicle loses in many cases the sensibility which it possesses in the normal state.

The swelling is hard, firm, not elastic; if pressed upon by the finger, the tumor conveys the sensation of a massive, fibro-cartilaginous, unelastic texture. The outer skin appears unaltered, keeps its natural color, remains cold, and can be moved to and fro over the swelling, to which it does not adhere. Only in a few cases some of the veins of the scrotum appear somewhat engorged.

Sarcocele, after it has reached a certain stage, is sometimes accompanied by hydrocele of the tunica vaginalis. This seems to be purely symptomatic, and is unaccompanied by fever or by any general derangement of the functions.

After the internal texture of the testicle has become disorganized, the seminal secretion gradually ceases, especially if both testes are diseased. The erections become less frequent and finally disappear altogether.

The physical properties of the semen undergo striking alterations in regard to quantity and consistence; the spermatozoa disappear, and, instead of semen, a transparent, almost watery fluid is secreted.

Syphilitic sarcocele may last months, and even several years. It never terminates in suppuration, nor does it ever transgress certain limits. After reaching a certain point, it here remains for a time, after which resolution takes place. This either takes place spontaneously, or in consequence of adequate treatment. Sometimes it happens that the testicle grows smaller in size; the patients consider this a good omen, endeavor to hasten the disease, but unfortunately this does not stop until the testicle has disappeared altogether.

In such a case other phenomena, which are generally met

with in eunuchs, supervene; for instance, the whole organism undergoes a change, the whole appearance and condition of the patient become altered, the voice loses its resonnance, etc.

There are cases where the disease takes a different turn; the swelling changes to a cartilaginous, fibrous and even osseous tumor. Ricord has seen several changes of this kind, and I have come across two such cases in my own practice.

Ricord has been led to believe by some cases that, if the vessels have not become atrophied, syphilitic sarcocele may terminate in simple resolution, and that the organ may again acquire its normal shape. We saw a case of this kind in his clinique; the patient died of inveterate syphilis, but a few months before his death, the testicle had resumed its natural shape and consistence.

According to Hamilton, syphilitic sarcocele only takes place from one to six years after the primary infection. He distinguishes two forms of the disease, the *simple syphilitic* and the *tuberculous syphilitic.* The former, he thinks, only befalls robust individuals, and is accompanied by secundary and tertiary symptoms, such as papulæ, pustules, scales, iritis, the lighter forms of ostitis and periostitis, etc. According to his statement the syphilitic tuberculous form is much more frequent than the former from which it differs in many essential particulars.

The penetrating Rokitansky, whose impartial and faithful investigations in pathological anatomy are of inestimable value for a correct knowledge of the diseased tissues, in reference to sarcocele, says: Chronic inflammation of the tunica albuginea and of the processes which it sends off towards the inner parts, occasions in rare cases only a considerable thickening of the fibrous membranes, material enlargement of the cellulo-fibrous tissue in the interior of the testicle, hypertrophy, a morbid hardness of the testicle, and finally atrophy." In reference to tuberculous syphilitic sarcocele, Rokitansky offers the following remarks: "Tuberculosis of the testicle principally affects young persons in consequence of excessive or unnatural gratification of the sexual passion; pathological anatomy has not yet succeeded in determining the connection of this disease with gonorrhœa; in other words, the blennorrhœic character of the constitutional disease and of the tubercle have not yet been proven, and the theory, that syphilitic sarcocele is an effect of gonorrhœa, lacks, in our estimation, an essential foundation. Tuberculosis of the testis generally developes itself in the shape of nodes, from the size of a millet seed to that of a pea, and coalescing into a shapeless mass, which scarcely ever terminates in resolution, but almost always in *suppuration*, and constitutes phthisis of the testicle. The increase of volume depends upon the number of tubercles and particularly upon the number of tuberculous groups, the tumor having an uneven, knotty surface. The tissue which surrounds the tubercle and its vomica, feels thick and callous, is dense, cartilaginous, resembling lard.

As in the lungs and pleural cavities, tuberculosis of the testicle is frequently accompanied by inflammation of the tunica albuginea leading to tuberculous deposits of a variety of shapes."

This shows that tuberculosis of the testis must be the result of a deeply-penetrating action of the syphilitic virus, and that there is an essential difference between gonorrhœal orchitis and syphilitic sarcocele.

As regards the causes and developments of syphilitic sarcocele, Ricord considers not only syphilis, but all other influences which act upon the testicle, as causes of this disease. Whatever exercises an irritating and exciting influence upon the testicles, may contribute to the development of sarcocele. Gonorrhœa contracted during the course of secondary syphilis, may excite the disease. Other causes, such as a contusion of these parts, a blow, excessive abstinence or else excessive indulgence, may likewise favor the development of sarcocele during secondary or tertiary syphilis. Sometimes the syphilitic dyscrasia is complicated with a cancerous, tuberculous, scrofulous diathesis; in such a case syphilitic sarcocele is likewise more easily developed.

11

Syphilitic sarcocele is found complicated with all sorts of disorganized secretions, such as: varicocele, hydrocele, which is quite frequent; acute and chronic gonorrhœal orchitis, simple orchitis, cysts and hydatids, and other forms of disorganizations.

The prognosis depends upon the simple or complicated nature of the disease. The less complicated the trouble, the sooner a gentle and rational treatment is instituted, the less the patient has been subjected to violent treatment: the more favorable the prognosis.

For syphilitic sarcocele, the following medicines have been found the most efficacious: *Calcarea carb.*, *Carbo veget.*, *Aurum*, *Kali carb.*, *Lycopod.* and *Spongia tosta.* But it may likewise be necessary to use one or more of the following remedies, according as they may be indicated by existing symptoms:

Acid. nitr., *Acid. phosph.*, *Alumina*, *Arsenicum*, *Belladonna*, *Baryt. mur.*, *Clemat.*, *China*, *Copaiva*, *Euphor.*, *Graphites*, *Lycopod.*, *Mercur. sol.*, *Mezerum*, *Oleander*, *Plumb. acet.*, *Pulsat.*, *Ranunc. bulb.*, *Rhodod.*, *Rhus tox.*

(The symptomatic indications for each of these remedies in particular imply a careful investigation and an accurate knowledge of the syphilitic disease from the beginning. In no other way would it be possible to arrive at a knowledge of the appropriate remedy in a case where sarcocele is apparently the only symptom, and may exist unaccompanied by any characteristic constitutional phenomena. An investigation of the whole series of symptoms constituting the syphilitic disease, will then first lead us to such remedies as *Acidum nitricum*, *Clematis*, *Copaiva*, *Mercurius sol.*, *Mercurius corrosivus*, *Mezereum*, which seem to be more closely related to the syphilitic virus.

Arsenicum, *China and Acidum phosphoricum*, *Plumbum acet.*, if the general constitution seems to be broken down, debilitated, the vital fluids seem to be tainted, or if the disease had been hastened by excesses;

Mercurius, *Clematis*, *Copaiv.*, *Pulsatilla*, if mismanaged gonorrhœa was either the immediate cause of the disease, or, at any rate, had complicated and aggravated it;

Belladonna, if symptoms of inflammatory congestion develope themselves in the tumor;

Graphites and Lycopodium, *Oleander* and *Belladonna*, if the disease is complicated with general scrofulosis, glandular swellings, chronic eruptions, as if it had grown worse and become more inveterate in consequence of the sudden suppression of a cutaneous eruption by a cold, washes, etc., in which latter case *Baryta mur.*, *Rhus tox.*, may be added to the last mentioned drugs.)

Induration of the corpora cavernosa of the penis.

This is one of the least known and least frequent phenomena of tertiary syphilis.

To our knowledge Ricord is the only author who has given an exact and correct description of this disease. He has observed some eighty cases, and, although the disease is very rare, yet he states that some eight or ten cases occur every year in his private or hospital practice. In our own practice, we have had a few cases of this disease to treat.

The induration of the corpora cavernosa generally developes itself in the following manner: In one or in both corpora cavernosa at the same time, the patient discovers, among other symptoms of tertiary syphilis, a small, hard body of the size of a grain of rice, which is, however, entirely painless. This hardness increases in size, either on one side, or on both sides at the same time, and may occur in the upper or lower portion or in the sides of the penis.

This disease runs a slow course, progresses very gradually, and is painless; but in proportion as the disease progresses, the penis deviates from its straight line in the following manner: If the induration is located on one side, the penis, if an erection takes place, will necessarily be turned towards the diseased side, where the erectile tissue has lost its dilatable character; this kind of erection, with the point of the penis turned towards the inguinal fold, has been termed, by Ricord, inguino-crural erection. If the induration is seated on the dorsum of the penis, the erection takes place upwards, the penis forming a curve with the concavity upwards and the glans turned towards the pubic arch. Ricord likewise saw the penis turned in other directions in consequence of an induration of the cavernous bodies; in some cases he saw it twisted like a ring.

[This affection never terminates in suppuration, and is frequently incurable. It is Ricord's opinion, though he does not give it as positive, that a violent gonorrhœa is, in most cases, the cause of this disease. In many cases the primary cause of the disease seemed to have been an act of violence committed while the penis was erect. He relates the case of a young student of medicine, where the disease seems to have resulted from a sudden apoplectic effusion of blood into the substance of the cavernous bodies. During a very violent erection the young man experienced an acute pain, apparently caused by a rupture of the cells, after which an effusion of blood took place, and coagula formed in the bodies, which could not be removed by absorption.

In this affection the following remedies will be found the most suitable to palliate, if not to cure, the disease:

Argent. nitr. Copaiva, Graphites, Hepar sulph., Mercur. acet., Mezer., Sabina.

In regard to symptomatic indications, we refer the reader to our remarks in the preceding paragraphs. The indications in the present case are the same. Not one of the remedies above mentioned can be said to be homœopathic to the disease upon purely symptomatic grounds, for an induration of the cavernous bodies of the penis has never been obtained by artificial drug-proving; the homœopathicity of the remedy to the disease in all such disorganizations must be traced back to the original conditions, to the starting-point of the disease, as well as to the starting-point of the drug-action; if these are alike, the remedy is homœopathic, and, if a cure be possible, and the medicine be properly used, a cure will undoubtedly be effected. All such disorganizations may, however, result from a complication of morbid miasms, syphilis, scrofulosis, tuberculosis and the like; and it may, therefore, be necessary to have recourse to more than one remedy during the treatment.

To the syphilitic and gonorrhœal dyscrasia correspond the *mercurial preparations: Argent. nit., Copaiv., Mezer., Thuja, Sabina, Acid. nitric., Pulsat., Canthar., Cannabis., Aurum, Silicea*, etc.

To the scrofulous and tuberculous dyscrasia: *Calcarea, Graphites, Lycop., Bellad., Arsenicum, Sulphur, Hepar sulph., China, Dulcamara*, etc.

In the case of hæmorrhage related above, the best remedy would undoubtedly have been *Aconite,* for the excessive erection was undoubtedly the result of an excessive congestion of the parts, and not the hæmorrhage a result of the erection.]

III. Tertiary Affections of the Periosteum and Bones.

These affections manifest themselves under four different forms, which, however, have to be regarded as different stages and terminations of the inflammatory process, but not as different forms of the syphilitic disease in the bones. These affections generally constitute the following successive series of phenomena; *syphilitic bone-pains* (dolores osteocopi,) *periostoses, exostoses* and *syphilitic necrosis and caries.*

Syphilitic bone-pains, dolores osteocopi.

These pains may be located in any portion of the osseous tissue, in the more deep-seated, as well as in the superficial layers, in the flat or long bones, in the articular extremities as well as in the shafts, and finally in the periosteum. There is not a single spot in the whole body that may not be affected by this pain. As a general rule, however, these pains occur most frequently in the superficial portions of the fibrous and osseous systems. Those portions of the bones which are less covered by the muscles and are more exposed to the open air, are most frequently invaded by syphilitic pains. Hence they occur more frequently in the tibia, radius, humerus, clavicle, sternum and in the bones of the skull, than in the more deep-seated bones. As a general rule, the compact portions of the bone are more frequently invaded by the pains than the spongy portions.

Bone-pains are to be numbered among the remotest manifestations of constitutional syphilis, and constitute in the true sense of the word tertiary phenomena. There is no case on record where bone-pains occurred, before five or six months after the primary chancre had elapsed. They may occur even ten, fifteen or twenty and even more years after the primary disease.

Bone-pains are most frequently caused by a sudden change in the weather. Although a sudden change from warm to cold weather favors the development of bone-pains, yet the inverse transition from cold to warmth, if the bone-pains are already developed, renders them much more acute. Hence it is, that they are very much aggravated when the patient goes to bed and begins to get warm. These nocturnal exacerbations of the bone-pains are exclusively attributable to the influence of the warmth of the bed. It is, therefore, wrong to consider the nocturnal exacerbations of the bone-pains a characteristic sign of their syphilitic character, and to term them *dolores nocturni*, as though they occurred preferably at night. Ricord states in reference to this subject, that these pains are felt at night only by those who go to bed at night, and get warm in the bed; but that they are not felt by those who spend the night in carousing; such persons only feel the pains in the day time while they are in bed and exposed to its warmth; in their case the pains would have to be called dolores diuturni. But they deserve neither one nor the other appellation, but simply increase by rest and the warmth of the bed, whether this occurs in the day time or at night. Ricord states, that among the rich who spend the summer in the country and the winter in the city, the bone-pains are felt at night in the summer, and in the day time in the winter; the reason of this is quite simple: in the winter the rich spend their nights in social entertainments and sleep in the day time, whereas, in the summer, they sleep at night and spend their days with fishing, hunting, riding on horse-back, and such like exercises.

In most cases, if the patients go to bed in the evening, the pains commence at eleven o'clock in the evening, and continue until two or three o'clock in the morning.

Syphilitic bone-pains always begin with a disagreeable sensitiveness. This gradually increases to a pain, until it finally changes to a frightful torture. It is peculiar to this pain to become seated in one spot of the bone, and always to reappear at the same place. The pain is aggravated by the least pressure, which is not the case when it is simply a rheumatic pain. After the pains have lasted for a time, they are not only excited by the warmth of the bed, but they are felt in the day time as well as at night, except that they are aggravated by rest. Syphilitic bone-pains may continue for a longer or shorter period without any alteration of the bone in the region where the pains are seated, becoming perceptible; they resemble neuralgic pains. Very often, however, these pains are the precursory symptoms of material changes of the bones which develope themselves speedily in some, and more tardily in other cases. Many patients experience these pains for months without perceiving any other change than a derangement of the reproductive functions and an increasing emaciation.

Syphilitic bone-pains most frequently terminate in periostosis.

The treatment is most efficaciously conducted by the following remedy:

Calcarea carbonica, *Carbo. animalis*, *Caustic.*, *Croc.*, *Fluor. ac.*, *Kali carb.*, *Laches.*, *Lycopod.*, *Magnes. carb.*, *Mercur. sol.*, *Mezer.*, *Natr. mur.*, *Nux vom.*, *Platin.*, *Plumb.*, *Plumb. acet.*, *Petrol.*, *Phosphor.*, *Pulsat.*, *Rhododend.*, *Staphys.*

[In regard to the special indications, we have to observe, that the principal remedies for this disease, provided the patient had not been saturated with mercury under allopathic treatment, are, 1, the *mercurial preparations*, *Merc. sol.*, *dulcis*, *corrosivus*, *ruber*, *acetatus*, etc.; 2, the *Hydriodate of potash*, if a good deal of mercury had been used, in which case it may be advisable to give the patient a few table-spoonfuls of an infusion of Sarsaparilla every day; 3, *Nitric acid*, and some of its compounds, such as the *Nitrate of potash*. In addition to these remedies, *Fluoric acid*, *Mezereum*, and *Staphysagria* may be employed, the two last named remedies more particularly, if the region where the pain is located feels sore, as if ulcerated.

Lachesis will be found useful, if the mercurial preparations had been employed to excess, or if mercury remains ineffectual under homœopathic treatment.

If there should be a complication with scrofulosis, and the patient should have been troubled in his childhood with weakness of the osseous system, rickets and such like diseases, we may select our medicines accordingly, and use for instance, *Calcarea carb.*, *Phosphor.* and *Phosphor. acidum*, *Pinus sylvestris*, likewise *China* and *Arsenic.*, the two latter more particularly if the constitution is shaken and requires building up.]

Periostitis syphilitica.

After the syphilitic bone-pains have continued for a length of time, alterations in the tissue of the periosteum begin to take place. The periosteum becomes inflamed, and exudations become distinctly perceptible when pressing upon the part. The exuded matter at first looks yellowish, of a gelatinous consistence, and, after a while, changes to a reddish or brownish fluid mixed with extravasated blood.

Syphilitic periostitis generally developes itself in the region where the pain had been felt. At this place we discover a rather circumscribed swelling of a greater or less extent, and with its base firmly adhering to the subjacent bone. The skin over this swelling is moveable, and its color seems unaltered. Gradually the swelling increases to the size of a pigeon's or hen's egg. The swelling is owing to the presence of the exuded matter between the periosteum and the bone, and resembling synovial fluid.

The swelling on first developing itself, is rather firm; it

does not fluctuate, but, when pressed upon, does not impart the sensation of a hard, resisting bone. Such swellings may increase to a considerable extent, but may likewise scatter without leaving a trace of their existence. A complete dispersion can only take place provided the exudation has not terminated in an actual disorganization. If no suitable treatment is instituted previous to such a result, an osseous degeneration (exostosis) is very apt to take place. Such osseous tumors arising from the consolidation of the plastic exudation, are termed *tophi*.

Periostitic inflammations resulting in exudations under the periosteum resembling the synovial fluid, are termed *gumma, gummata*.

Exostosis.

These swellings are always preceded by periostitis, and do not develope themselves until the bone-pains have lasted for a time. They run a very slow course. They arise from an osseous disorganization of the plastic exudation in periostitis, a disorganization which takes place in a similar manner as the callus in the fracture of bones. The morbid process commences partially in the periosteum and in the superficial layer of the compact bony substance which is thickened by an additional layer of osseous exudation between the bone and the periosteum. On its surface the exudation is cartilaginous; the deeper layers exhibit an osseous consistence. After the exudation has lasted for a time, it acquires throughout the consistence of bone, and is of various thickness. At first the surface of the swelling is rough, sometimes as if covered with warts; the older the swelling, and the more it acquires the consistence of ivory, the more its surface becomes smooth and even.

These rather superficial exostoses are of various shapes; sometimes they form a flat, extensive layer, resembling a simple distension or swelling of the original bone; at other times the exostoses constitute fusiform, pad-shaped, round or prominent, knotty, and even pedunculated tumors.

In other cases the exostosis commences in the interior of the bony substance, or on the inner surface adjoining the diploë or marrow. The exudation taking place within the bony substance, the bone grows thicker and harder; the tumor which encroaches upon, and sometimes fills up entirely the hollow interior, acquires the consistence of ivory, and, on its outer surface, represents a flat, round elevation. Sometimes, several of such exostoses are placed side by side, at first isolated, but afterwards coalescing. In the commencement of the disease, the patients do not complain of any pain except the bone-pains. These continue often for a long period before the exostosis shows itself, and abate as soon as the bone begins to swell. The exostosis never terminates in suppuration, nor does it even become carious. It either remains unaltered during the patient's life-time, or a gradual reduction is effected by suitable treatment, sometimes after the tumor had been in existence for years. An exostosis may arise in a locality where it may give origin to a variety of distressing secondary phenomena. Large exostoses on the lower extremities impede motion, and render it painful, interfere with the functions of the muscles and tendons, and may lead to atrophy of the part. Exostoses on the inner surface of the skull may cause all that train of phenomena consequent upon pressure of the brain and of its membranes such as paralysis, spasms and so forth.

The following remedies will be found the most adequate to the complete or partial reduction of syphilitic periostoses and exostoses:

Asafœtida, Aurum, Bryon., China, Conium, Mercur. sol., Mezer., Phosphor., Ruta, Sabina, Sepia, Silicea, Sulphur, Stannum, Staphysagria, Thuja.

[To these remedies we should add the hydriodate of potash.

Aurum, Phosphorus, and the *phosphate of lime,* also *Ruta,* seem to be particularly adapted to exostoses of the cranium; the two last named remedies more particularly if the syphilitic dyscrasia is complicated by scrofulosis.

Asafœtida, Mercurius, the *Hydriodate of potash, Staphy-*

sagria and *Silicea,* will be found particularly useful in exostoses of the long or hollow bones.

Thuja and *Sabina* refer more especially to a sycosic character of the tumor.

Acidum nitricum and the *hydriodate of potash* are suitable remedies when we have reason to suspect a complication of mercurial and syphilitic dyscrasia.

The *mercurial preparations* are undoubtedly the principal remedy for this disorganization, and the treatment may safely be commenced with them, provided mercury had not been previously administered in allopathic doses; and even then, small homœopathic doses of mercury, if judiciously administered, may be of great use in this disease.

Ledum palustre may be given for hard tubercles and tophi in the joints. The mercurial preparations are likewise indicated for this affection, if accompanied with arthritic pains in the joints.

Rhus tox. is another remedy for swelling of bones, if the parts are painful and the pain is worse during rest than during motion, with a sense of paralytic numbness and weakness in the parts.

Sulphur has likewise been used with advantage for swelling and curvature of the bones.]

Syphilitic caries and necrosis.

We have seen that syphilitic periostoses and exostoses result from a specific inflammation of the periosteum and of the bone. They may be considered as terminations of periostitis and ostitis, in the one case in *resolution,* in the other in *induration.* A third termination of ostitis is *suppuration.* This is the most pernicious, but fortunately the least frequent of all the terminations of ostitis. In compact bones, of low vitality, the inflammatory process generally terminates in exostosis, much less frequently in suppuration.

In bones endowed with a higher degree of vitality, if the patients are sickly, and the osseous system is disposed to inflammatory conditions, syphilis will more readily lead to caries and necrosis. Hence the spongy tissue of bones is more easily attacked with caries and necrosis than the denser tissue.

The termination in suppuration takes place in the following manner: the diseased part is exceedingly painful. The pains continue day and night, only that at night the pains are much more violent. The pain has the general character of just such a pain as is experienced previous to the suppurative process setting in. First it is aching, tensive, afterwards throbbing, and increases in proportion as the suppuration is drawing near. Soon after the soft parts commence to change, they coalesce with the tumor. At first this is circumscribed and resisting, afterwards it becomes fluctuating. The abscess does not always open in the region where the part is diseased; the pus may burrow downwards between the muscular layers; the skin over the tumor becomes inflamed and breaks spontaneously, unless opened, in several places. At first fistulous abscesses form, all which lead to the denuded bone. Afterwards the pustules run together into a larger abscess, at the bottom of which the carious bone either lies exposed, or is partially covered by rapidly suppurating, lardaceous layers, and afterwards by adventitious granulations. The surrounding skin is quite red, and, together with the subjacent parts, unites with the bone in one compact mass. With the suppuration and destruction of the soft parts, the vitality of the bone gets lost, the calcareous portions are laid bare, so that the dead calcareous mass alone remains. This dead matter acts, in its turn, like a foreign body, and helps to keep up the suppurative process. But there are cases where the suppuration penetrates through the osseous tissues, and the bony mass becomes decomposed. In the one case the bones begin to die as soon as the destruction of the soft parts commences; in the other case the bone becomes ichorous, and is decomposed into larger or smaller pieces. The former disorganization is termed *necrosis*, the latter *caries*. These two disorganizations are frequently found united.

Although any part of the osseous system may be marked by caries, yet this disorganization befalls principally the bones of the cranium, those of the face, and more particularly the upper maxillary bones. It occurs very rarely in the submaxillary bone. The palatine bones are frequently attacked. In many cases the affection commences in the corners of the nose and the caries of the palatine bones is the result of the affection of the adjoining soft parts, in consequence of which the bones become denuded. Very frequently the carious perforations of the the palatine bones are caused by perforating tubercles of the nasal bones. The dental portion of the maxillary bones is most frequently attacked by caries. The parts which constitute the sockets of the teeth, swell, and these more or less painful swellings are followed by abscesses which raise the soft parts, and the fetid odor of caries emanates from the suppurating disorganization. After the breaking of the abscesses, the probe soon reveals the rough surface of a carious bone. Afterwards, on examining the teeth, it will be found that one tooth alone cannot be shaken, but that, upon endeavoring to shake several teeth together, the whole dental portion of the jaw is moved. If this motion is distinctly perceptible, the bone is dead, and there is no hope remaining of preserving it or reducing it to its normal condition. The ascending processes of the palate-bones generally remain free from caries; on the contrary the nasal cartilages are principally invaded by this disease; the vomer which has a denser tissue, becomes necrotic; the nose caves in, the outer nasal bones are not destroyed, but the form of the nose becomes nevertheless altered.

The bones of the cranium are likewise frequently attacked by syphilitic caries and necrosis.

Syphilitic caries and necrosis of the jaw leads to the loss of teeth, indistinctness of speech in consequence of the perforation of the palatine vault.

If the disorganization affects the nose, the loss of a few cartilages may not be attended with any considerable inconvenience. But if the vomer and the other cartilages of the nose should be destroyed, the nose will cave in, and the shape of the face will become considerably altered. The destructive process likewise invades the septum; the nose forms only *one* cavity; the Schneiderian membrane becomes altered and covered with a pseudo-plastic layer which secretes a peculiar, fetid matter; some portions of the Schneiderian membrane remain sound. The matter which is secreted in the nose, adheres; it is not expelled as readily as the common nasal mucus, and it accumulates in large quantity. There is a secretion of purulent, ichorous matter continually going forward, having a sickly, nauseous odor.

Caries and necrosis of the skull-bones are likewise of frequent occurrence. This condition is so much the more important as it may lead to dangerous cerebral affections. If the external plate is diseased, the cerebral functions remain undisturbed, except the pain. But the thing is different, if the tumor is seated on the vitreous table; in such a case violent headache, vertigo, tremor, numbness of the limbs, and, after a period, semilateral paralysis of the muscles of the face and remainder of the head, delirium and epileptiform convulsions may supervene. Caries of the frontal and parietal bones leads to inflammation and ulceration of the meningeal membranes. Caries of the frontal bones results in perforation of the frontal sinuses, destruction of the cribriform plate and of the adjoining parts.

In caries and necrosis the following remedies will be found useful:

Asafœtida, Aurum, Argentum nitricum, Baryta carb., Bellad., Bryonia, Calcarea carb., Caustic., China, Conium, Dulcam., Mercur. sol., Mezer., Nux vom., Phosphorus, Pulsat., Rhus tox., Sabina, Silicea, Staphys., Sulphur.

[To this list we may add:

Tartar emetic, frictions with which, upon the skull, have produced caries of the skull-bones, and which may therefore be supposed possessed of curative virtues in this disease.

Mercurius solub., has cured caries of the bones in general, and caries of the joints, of the auricula auris, and of the maxillary bone in particular.

Mezereum has cured caries of the bones.

Calcarea phosphorata is useful in caries, also caries of the skull.

Aurum foliatum is a great remedy for caries of the facial bones, nasal bones and palate.

Hepar sulphuris in caries of the hip-joint, or in caries produced by abuse of mercury, for which *Aurum* and *Silicea* will likewise be found indicated.

Silicea has cured caries of the humerus, jaw-bone, malar-bone, tibia, and vertebræ.

Calcarea carbon. is useful in caries of the vertebræ.

Cistus canadensis has been found of great use in caries of the lower jaw, and of the facial bones; in the latter case it was used as an infusion internally, and in the shape of a poultice externally.

China, *Conium* and *Sulphur* are adapted to mercurial, scrofulous and syphilitic caries.

Asafœtida will likewise be found useful in mercurial and scrofulous caries, although this remedy is generally much less valuable than is supposed.]

IV. Tertiary Affections of the Muscles and Tendons.

Ricord terms these affections syphilitic contractions of the muscles and tendons, and ranks them among the most curious phenomena of tertiary syphilis. They are exceedingly rare, and generally attack persons of advanced age who had been syphilitic and exposed to repeated rains and colds.

The syphilitic affections of the muscles and tendons begin with pains which are very similar to bone-pains, have intermissions like these, and are generally made worse by the warmth of the bed. Being considerably aggravated by motion, these pains have also been termed syphilitic rheumatism. Even after the pains have lasted only a short period, a permanent contraction of the muscles takes place. The distortion of the limb caused by such contractions, developes itself very slowly. In general the disease runs a slow course. In the region where the pain is located, the patient gradually experiences a sort of rigidity, a difficulty of motion, especially when attempting to stretch the part; for then the muscle feels as if it were contracted. Little by little such a contraction really takes place; the limb remains permanently bent. The contraction never takes place suddenly as if caused by some sudden nervous derangement. The starting-point of this contraction is not to be sought in the brain or spinal column, but in the substance of the muscle itself and in the alteration which the tissue undergoes. Coagulable lymph exudes between the muscular fibres, forming after a longer or shorter period a fibrous, cartilaginous and even osseous disorganization, which results in atrophy of the part. The skin covering these muscular disorganizations is moveable, and not at all altered in appearance. The neighboring lymphatic glands frequently swell. A change in the weather causes pain in the muscular swelling.

Such muscular disorganizations generally take place in the flexor muscles of the forearm, in the muscles of the eye, in the sterno-cleido-mastoideus muscles, in the posterior cervical muscles, especially the transversalis colli; in the pectoralis major, the gluteus maximus, and in the gastrocnemius muscle. These muscles and the corresponding parts become contracted.

The tongue and lips are likewise liable to such contractions. In the tongue the exudation generally takes place in a portion of the hypoglossus muscle only, very seldom in the whole substance of the muscle. The tongue is swollen, the tumor is hard and seated within the substance of the tongue where it constitutes a more or less circumscribed, globular elevation, which is exceedingly sensitive to motion. Talking, chewing and even swallowing are impeded. This affection is frequently confounded with cancer, not to the benefit of the patient. In this affection there are never any lancing pains, nor is the surface of the tongue indurated or warty as in cancer.

Syphilitic affections of the tendons are more frequent than

those of the muscles. They are characterized by circumscribed, hard, rounded or irregularly-shaped thickenings, which are painful only at the commencement. These tendinous swellings are likewise occasioned by exudations in the sheath or in the substance of the tendons, which at first are liquid, gradually become organised, and afterwards acquire a calcareous consistence. The swelling constitutes a perceptible prominence on the tendon, and, if situated on tendons adjoining the skin, as in the palm of the hand, in the wrist-joint, on the tendo Achilles, the skin and the swelling coalesce; a few bunches only are perceptible to the touch.

For tertiary affections of the muscles and tendons, the following remedies will be found most appropriate:

Angustura spur., Aconit., Alum., Ammon. carb., Acidum nitr., Arsen. Ammon. mur., Bellad., Baryt. carb., Berber., Coccul., Crot., Caust., Colch., Carb. animalis, Euphorb., Euphras., Graphit., Guajac., Hyoscyamus, Ignat., Indigo, Kreosot., Laches., Lycop., Mercur. sol., Natr. mur., Nux vom., Opium, Oleand., Plumb. acet., Petrol. Ranunc. bulb., Rhus tox., Sabina, Secale., Sarsap., Sepia, Spigelia, Stramon., Silicea, Spongia, Sulph., Thuja, Veratr., Zincum.

[Among this large number of remedies we have to distinguish

1. Such as refer to purely syphilitic condition.

2. Such as refer to syphilitic conditions complicated with rheumatism.

3. Such as refer to a complication of syphilis and scrofulosis; and

4. Such as correspond to syphilis complicated with general debility.

Among the first class we number *Acidum nitricum, Kali hydriodicum, Mercurius sol., Sabina, Thuja;* the two last named particularly, when the affection can be traced to sycosis.

To the second class belong *Aconite, Belladonna, Colchicum, Guajacum, Mercurius solub., Nux vom., Sepia, Sulphur;*

Aconite and *Belladonna* being principally indicated when inflammatory symptoms are present, the swellings feel hot and sore, and the least attempt to extend the parts causes pain.

Guajacum is more particularly indicated when the posterior muscles of the legs are the seat of the disease, with lancinations from the feet upwards.

Mercurius, when the parts are stiff and ache, without the pain being very acute ; the patient feels chilly when exposed to the least breath of air.

Colchicum may be used if Aconite seemed indicated but did not produce the desired effect, or it may be given in alternation with Aconite, especially if the derangement was caused by exposure to wet or a draught of air ; Rhus tox. is likewise indicated in this disease.

Sepia and *Sulphur* are more particularly adapted to chronic forms of this disease.

The third class comprises the following remedies : *Aconite*, *Belladonna*, *Baryt. carb.*, *Graphit.*, *Lycopod.*, *Sarsap.*, *Silic.*, *Spongia* and *Sulphur*.

Belladonna, Spongia, and Sulphur may be used first in preference to the other medicines, not omitting, however, the exhibition of the mercurial preparations which cannot be dispensed with in any form of the disease.

If the syphilitic affection is accompanied with a general sinking or debility of the constitution, we may use the remedies mentioned in the fourth division, principally *Arsenicum*, *Baryta*, *Carbo. anim.*, *China*, *Ignatia*, *Oleander*, *Plumbum acet.*, *Sepia*, *Veratrum*, although any of the other medicines may likewise be indicated.]

V. Tertiary Affections of the Eyes.

Beside the iritis syphilitica which Ricord numbers among the secondary affections of the eyes, he speaks of tertiary affections of these organs, which have never been mentioned before by any author.

Tertiary affections may either involve the eye itself, or its appendages, or the neighboring parts. These affections may occur alone without any other part of the body being diseased. Ricord treated patients for diplopia in whom, after death, the muscles of the eye were found altered in the same manner as other muscles are. Most patients whose eyes are affected in this manner have an excellent vision; but as soon as they look upwards or sideways, every thing appears to them double; this alteration of the visual functions occurs quite suddenly, and ceases again as soon as the original direction of the eye is restored. In some cases the muscles of the eye were contracted to such an extent that the patient squinted. Ricord treated one patient for strabismus convergens, the outer muscles having their natural mobility and length. According to this physician the most frequent contractions occur in the inferior rectus muscle, in consequence of which the eyeball may be permanently drawn downwards out of its horizontal axis.

Beside these contractions of the muscles of the eyes, there are alterations of the visual functions arising from syphilitic affections of the sclerotica. This membrane may, like the other fibrous portions of the body, undergo alterations of tissue which exercise an important influence upon the shape and functions of the eye. Alterations of the nervous structure of the eye may likewise lead to amaurosis. Ricord relates several cases of amblyopia occasioned by tertiary syphilis, and the same author gives it as his opinion that lenticular or capsular cataract may likewise arise from the action of the syphilitic miasm upon the lens or its enveloping membrane.

The following remedies may be of use in the treatment of these affections of the eye:

Alum., *Agaric.*, *Ammon. carb.*, *Arsenic.*, *Aurum*, *Baryt. carb.*, *Bellad.*, *Con.*, *Digit.*, *Euphorb.*, *Graphit.*, *Hyosc.*, *Iod.*, *Nitr. acid.*, *Petrol.*, *Pulsat.*, *Secale*, *Stram.*, *Veratr.*

[For contraction of the muscles of the eye, we may use: *Aconite*, *Belladonna* and the more penetrating mercurial preparations such as *Mercurius corrosivus, dulcis, ruber.*

For disorganizations of the lens and membranes of the eye, *Belladonna*, *Arsenicum*, *Acidum nitr.*, *Cannabis*, *Iodine*, may be given.

For alterations of the nervous functions, we have *Belladonna*, *Conium*, *Digitalis*, *Hyoscyamus*, *Stramonium*, *Tussiiago petasites.*]

VI. Tertiary Affections of the Nerves and Central Nervous Organs.

Syphilis may affect the brain and spinal marrow idiopathically. Alterations of the meningeal membranes, after the bones of the cranium or of the vertebral column have been destroyed by syphilis, must necessarily affect the functions of the brain or spinal column, but these derangements would not be idiopathic. It is Ricord's opinion that the syphilitic poison affects directly the nervous centres. In the brain of persons who had died of syphilis, he found tubercles which bore great resemblance to syphilitic deposits in other parts of the body. Such tubercles in the brain or spinal marrow must of course produce marked alterations in the cerebral or nervous functions during the life-time of the patient, And it is indeed true that the motor and sentient powers of syphilitic patients are affected in a manner which can only be traced to syphilis.

One of the most frequent disturbances of both the motor and sentient nerves is paraplegia. Ricord gives it as his opinion, that syphilis is a very frequent cause of general paralysis or paraplegia. It is only recently, that the discovery was made, that syphilis may cause a paralysis of the seventh pair of nerves. In the "*Deutsche Klinik*," Knorre relates several cases of paralysis caused by syphilis, which he treated in the Hamburgh hospital; among them two cases of paralysis of the facial nerve, and several cases of diplopia and amaurosis.

Epilepsy and catalepsy are likewise caused by tertiary syphilis. Ricord relates the case of one of the most distinguished actors of Paris whom he treated some years ago for syphilitic epilepsy. This gentleman had been treated in vain by a number of the most distinguished physicians of Paris; Ricord undertook an anti-syphilitic course of treatment, and removed the attacks in some months.

We must not forget to mention a peculiar derangement of the nervous system caused by syphilis, and which is undoubtedly noticed by every practitioner; Ricord terms it *syphiliphobia.* This is one of the worst forms of hypochondria. Without a single sign of syphilis being perceptible any where in the patient's constitution, he nevertheless fancies that he is affected with the disease. This imaginary syphilis is a fixed idea with such patients; it does not leave them by day or by night; the least spot, pustule, pain, is a symptom of syphilis. Such patients are a perfect burthen to themselves, to others, and particularly to their physician; they come to him for every little trifle, show him their tongues, ask him to examine their private parts or the interior of the throat; the least redness and secretion of mucous causes them great trouble, and confirms them in their apprehensions. They examine themselves in the looking-glass, look at their tongues, and feel unhappy if they discover a few small papillæ, or if the orifice of the Stenonian duct excites their attention. In this way they go about, physicking themselves as advised either by quacks or physicians, until their constitution is ruined.

We have found the following remedies the most efficacious in derangements of the nervous functions from syphilitic causes:

Acid. nitr., *Anacard.*, *Angust.*, *Arnica*, *Arsenicum*, *Bryon.*, *China*, *Cocculus*, *Colchicum*, *Nux vom.*, *Oleander*, *Plumb.*, *Plumb. acet.*, *Sepia*, *Silicea*, *Stannum*, *Zincum*.

[*Anacardium* will be found particularly useful when the functions of the special senses, and the intellectual functions are impaired;

Angustura for cramps, spasms of the spinal marrow, especially when of a tetanic nature;

Arnica, *Arsenicum* and *China*, when the patient complains of debility, the flesh becomes flabby, looks sickly and sallow, the appetite is poor, sleep disturbed, the reproductive functions are declining;

Nux vomica, for derangement of the sentient functions, numbness and creeping in the extremities, spasmodic twitchings, constipation, load at the stomach;

Plumbum acet., atrophied condition of the extremities, paralysis, dulness of the mental powers;

Iodine, for a similar condition as Plumbum.

Zincum, general emaciation, colliquative discharges, chronic headache, sleeplessness.]

VII. Tertiary Affections of the Parenchymatous Organs and Syphilitic Cachexia.

We have shown in the course of this work, that the first tendency of syphilis is to the skin and mucous membranes; as it progresses it invades the fibrous membranes, the bones, muscles, tendons, and even nerves. These different organs are liable to the most horrible disorganizations from the syphilitic virus, in consequence of which the organism is sadly and frightfully undermined. But the destructive process goes much farther, and even invades the parenchymatous organs of the interior cavities. Until recently, these syphilitic affections of the inner organs were little heeded and even unsuspected. And yet many deep-seated affections of the liver, larynx, lungs, and even the heart and brain, are enkindled by the syphilitic poison.

Professor Dittrich, of Erlangen, was the first who instituted extensive inquiries into the syphilitic affections of the liver, and communicated the results of his inquiries in the "*Prager Vierteljahrschrift.*" According to his observations, the substance of the liver is never wholly, but only partially attacked by the syphilitic process which consists in partially organized exudations caused by inflammatory action. These inflammations are usually cured, only leaving cicatrices behind. Without giving any further account of the distinguished pathologico anatomical investigations of the Professor, we will simply state that the further progress of the disease in the liver leads to suppuration of this organ.

Not only the liver, but also the spleen, kidneys and even the thyroid gland are involved in this process, which ultimately leads to dropsy and death. Such morbid alterations of parenchymatous organs constitute the remotest forms of constitutional syphilis.

A syphilitic derangement of the liver announces itself in the first place by jaundice, bloating of the liver, disposition to diarrhœa and derangement of the digestive functions ; afterwards the syphilitic cachexia which we shall describe more completely hereafter, develope themselves. It is undoubtedly true, that the abuse of mercury aggravates the affections of the liver. The process of exudation which is going on in the liver, excites inflammations, swellings and sanguineous engorgements of the liver, and, if the enveloping membranes of the liver are inflamed, a dangerous local or general peritonitis may ensue. A general syphilitic cachexia winds up the malady. The skin becomes sallow, livid or yellowish. The fat vanishes, the muscles grow thinner, the strength fails, and even sight and hearing grow weaker; the process of sanguification is altered, and a state of anæmia and hydræmia, with their consequences, such as dropsy, etc., set in. The blood-disks are less in number. These phenomena of a disturbed reproduction of the blood are accompanied by palpitation of the heart, murmurs in the arteries, and chlorotic symptoms. In some cases, intermittent or remittent fevers, disposition to sanguineous extravasations under the skin (scurvy, purpura hæmorrhagica, etc.,) effusions of blood into the lungs, bowels, interior of the bones; atheromatous processes in the larger arteries and lastly dropsy supervene.

Since his first communications, Professor Dittrich has published a new series of observations, and has added new reasons for the confirmation of his views.

The cases which came under his notice, were divided by him into three groups, the first of which confirmed the co-existence of an inflammatory process in the liver and loss of substance of the vault of the palate and of the fauces.

The second group contained four cases without any apparent affection of the fauces, but with sufficient symptoms of a syphilitic diathesis to permit one to ascribe the affection of the liver to the previous action of the syphilitic virus. He likewise directs attention to the exudations into the substance of the lungs, which were characterized by similar symptoms as the exudations into the substance of the liver, whence the Professor concludes that the pulmonary exudations are likewise of syphilitic origin.

In the third group we have two cases where the exudative process in the liver, and the transformation of the exuded fluid into pus, still exist in their original form. From the fact that some portions of the liver are already cicatrized, whilst new exudations are going on in other portions, the Professor argues the chronic character of the exudation.

Ricord has shown with a good deal of accuracy that similar morbid proccsses may be going on in the lungs. A considerable number of post-mortem examinations have led him to the opinion that there are pulmonary affections which have to be charged upon the presence of syphilitic tubercles. It is true Ricord has arranged this morbid process side by side with syphilitic tubercles or gummata of the outer skin. These adventitious growths run the same course in the lungs as in any other portion of the body; the swelling has the same form, runs the same course, and likewise terminates in suppuration. The patients raise pus, the same as in the last stage of phthisis tuberculosa; they grow thin, feeble, and soon die from this extreme derangement of the respiratory functions.

A development of the syphilitic tubercle may involve the neighboring parts. For instance, if the palatine vault or the Schneiderian membrane should be affected, the adjoining bones and cartilages may become involved in the disorganization. This may lead to syphilitic perichondritis and to syphilitic laryngitis and syphilitic phthisis of the larynx. We have had several cases of this destructive malady to treat. Porter,

Hasse, Albers, Jansen and Rokitansky, all mention this disease, and Rokitansky moreover attributes it to the action of mercury. According to Dittrich the laryngeal disease is not a form of genuine primary perichondritis, but an affection that first invades the soft parts, and gradually induces a syphilitic stricture of the larynx (laryngosthenosis.) A portion of the exudation or even the whole of it, changes to a fibrous, callous growth, encroaching upon the internal space of the larynx. Sometimes a portion of the exudation changes to pus, forming ulcers of various shapes and dimensions. If a deep-seated portion of the exudation, which is in contact with the cartilage of the larynx, should change to pus, the destruction of the cartilage and necrosis of this organ become unavoidable, and abscesses round the laryngeal cartilages are the natural result.

Ricord states that he saw tubercles in a heart, some of which were about to soften. Similar tubercles were seen in the lungs of this same individual, and on the skin some of the same kind of tubercles were already softened. There had not been any symptoms of genuine tubercular phthisis in this patient, previous to his contracting syphilis; it seemed, therefore, rational to attribute the presence of tubercles in his case to the action of the syphilitic virus.

Accordingly Ricord advises whenever we have to deal with inexplicable, deep seated, mysterious, disguised derangements of the functions, and there is the least reason to suppose that the trouble arises from syphilitic taint, to institute an anti-syphilitic treatment. He thinks that if this course had been pursued, a pretty fair number of consumptive patients might have been saved.

The following remedies either cure or palliate this disease:

Acid. nitr., *Acid. phosph.*, *Arsen.*, *Alumina*, *Bryon.*, *Carbo. animal.*, *Carbo. veget.*, *Calcar. carb.*, *China*, *Chin. sulph.*, *Iodine*, *Kali carbon.*, *Lactura vicosa*, *Lycopod.*, *Mercur. viv.*, *Mercur. sol.*, *Mercur. dulc.*, *Nux moschat.*, *Plumb.*, *Plumb. acet.*, *Sabad.*, *Secale*, *Sepia*, *Sulphur*, *Thuja.*

[Particular indications for each of these remedies are of course interesting and important, but the symptoms are so various that it seems almost impossible to furnish a complete list of the symptomatic characteristics to which each of these remedies corresponds. We will therefore content ourselves with the principal outlines of each remedy, and refer the reader to the symptomen-codex.

Acidum nitricum: Signs of a general decomposition of the fluids; scorbutic symptoms in the mouth; ptyalism; foul ulcers of the gums and tongue; bleeding of the gums; ulcerative soreness of the hairy scalp; falling off of the hair; difficulty of hearing; humming and roaring in the ears; ulceration of the nose with yellow and fetid discharge; ulcers in the throat with putrid smell from the mouth; costiveness, with dampness and itching of the anus; scraping sensation in the larynx with dryness and hoarseness, also cough with expectoration of black coagulated blood; weakness of the extremities; soreness and lameness of the joints; anxious dreams at night; blotches and boils on the skin; sallowness of the skin; spasms and epilepsy.

Phosphori acidum may be used for symptoms similar to the former, especially when there is a complication of symptoms arising from loss of animal fluids, onanism; the joints are more particularly involved; humid, itch-like eruptions on the forehead, face, back, thighs; inveterate ulcers secreting a bad pus, with shaggy borders and a burning and stinging pain; the lungs seem invaded by the syphilitic process, with dry cough, also bloody cough.

Arsenicum: General sinking of strength; bloating, as if dropsical; scaly; also malignant eruptions or ulcerations; fetid diarrhœa, or exhausting bloody diarrhœic stools with constant and distressing urging; pale face; jaundiced color of the skin; trembling of the limbs; arthritic and rheumatic pains in the limbs diminished by moving the parts.

Carbo veget. may be used, if Arsenic. should not procure the relief intended, and more particularly if symptoms of dyspepsia, acidity of the stomach, palpitation of the heart, are present. In such a case

Carbo animalis may be tried, instead of vegetabilis.

Iodine corresponds to glandular disorganizations, atrophied conditions of the extremities, mercurial complications.

Mercurius sol. and *dulcis:* disorganizations of the tonsils, ulceration of the throat, mouth, skin, bone-pains, especially in bed, and more particularly about the skull, with excessive painfulness of the hairy scalp; costiveness, dry, hard, and lumpy stool, urine depositing a chalk-like and purulent sediment.

Plumbum acet: Melancholy mood, emaciation, debility, anguish about the heart, flaccidity and paleness of the muscles, hectic fever, ptyalism.

Sulphur: Itch-like eruptions, ulcers on the tibia, mercurial complications, ptyalism, bleeding of the gums, tumors in the joints of the arms and feet.

Thuja: Syphilitic dyscrasia, characterized by condylomatous excrescenses with a broad base, discharging pus and blood; pressure in the region of the bones, here and there, accompanied by a pricking, scraping sensation; headache as if a button were pressed against the skull.

For syphilitic perichondritis, the best remedies are: *Belladonna, Hepar sulphuris, Drosera, Spongia, Causticum.*

Drosera and *Spongia* are particularly adapted to a dry, spasmodic cough, principally troublesome at night.

Kali bichromicum, if the cough is accompanied with ulcerative pains in the region of the larynx, and raising of pus from the painful spot.

Causticum, when the weakness in the larynx is characterized by permanent hoarseness and weakness of speech.]

Syphilis of little Children.

Constitutional syphilis may be transmitted by the father or mother to the fetus, but it is very rare that infants are infected by the mother during the passage of the child through the vagina.

In congenital syphilis the primary ulcers are wanting; however, the disease exercises considerable influence upon the fetus in the uterus, and a large number of syphilitic mothers either miscarry or their children are still-born. This is especially the case where both parents are affected by the disease. The still-born infant exhibits all the traces of a deeply-rooted syphilis. Weakly children born at full term, or premature children die either during or shortly after their expulsion from the womb. Many children tainted with congenital syphilis seem to be robust and healthy at birth. A few days or weeks elapse before syphilitic symptoms are perceived. But at the expiration of two or three weeks, and in rare cases, of the second month, the first signs of the disease make their appearance.

Children affected with congenital syphilis, are uneasy even a few days after their birth; they cry day and night, emaciate very rapidly, their face looks old and withered, and their eyes are sunken. Soon after there appear in the region of the sexual organ, groins, on the thighs, heels, buttocks, round the anus, and even in the umbilical region, and sometimes all over the skin, circumscribed spots of a bright copper color, rising speedily above the skin in the shape of blotches, and sometimes running together, especially at the soles of the feet, and covering them entirely. The same phenomenon soon after developes itself on the palms of the hands. Simultaneously a papulous eruption, which afterwards changes to small, dirty-yellow pustules surrounded with a broad areola, breaks out on the chest, back, in the face, and on the hairy scalp. On the inflamed portions of the feet, hands and anus, tuberculous elevations start up, which become covered with blisters resembling pemphigus; these blisters change to excoriations and afterwards to deep ulcers, particularly between the toes, on the heels, in the inguinal folds, at the perinæum and in the axillæ. At the anus ulcerated rhagades develope themselves.

In spite of the characteristic nature of these phenomena, mothers seldom pay much attention to them unless they should have become quite serious. They generally look upon these symptoms as common soreness, and employ such common domestic remedies as the nurse or some old woman may advise. Sometimes the eruption disappears without any medical treatment. Frequently, however, superficial ulcers in the corners of the mouth and in the nose show themselves. The child is attacked with a discharge from the nose which at first looks like catarrh. Gradually the discharge increases, the conjunctiva and especially the margin of the eyes, the Meibomian glands become inflamed and suppurate. The ulcers in the corners of the mouth penetrate more deeply, their edges become raised and red. The voice sounds hoarse, thin and moaning. Hæmorrhage from the mouth and nose sets in; the latter is frequently stopped up with crusts, by which the nursing is rendered difficult; the breathing is accompanied by a slight rattling. the head breaks out, and some of the lymphatic glands swell. Ulcers break out in the fauces, deglutition becomes painful, the voice has a peculiar, hoarse sound. Such children seldom live longer than one year, for the syphilitic disease becomes complicated with acute tuberculosis of the brain. If the child does not perish in this manner, the syphilitic cachexia developes itself. The child becomes chlorotic, the skin assumes a dirty gray-yellow color like wax, a complete state of anæmia developes itself, the reproductive system is prostrate, and the child dwindles down to a skeleton. Not unfrequently these symptoms assume the form of scrophulosis, or chronic hydrocephalus developes itself. Congenital syphilis in children, generally runs a very rapid course, and, unless speedily arrested by proper treatment, terminates fatally.

If the infection dates from the passage of the child through the vagina, or if it took place while the child was nursing—the former is supposed to take place during slow labor—the above-mentioned eruption is principally seen on parts where the skin is delicate and deprived of the cheesy covering, namely, the neck and the sexual parts; the course of this form of the disease is the same as that of congenital syphilis.

Cazenave does not admit the possibility of congenital syphilis. He points out the fact that there is perhaps not a single well authenticated case of syphilis communicated to the child during its passage through the vagina. He believes, however, in the possibility of syphilis being transmitted to a child by the influence of the milk, and while at the breast. Moreover, he thinks that the disease is much more frequently inherited from the father than from the mother.

According to this same author, the syphilides of nurses are exceedingly injurious to children.

In little children, affected with congenital syphilis, Wallace has seen a peculiar cutaneous disease, of which no mention has yet been made any where, and which he describes as follows:

There appear on various parts of the body, especially on the back, isolated papulæ of the size of peas and rather hard; they remain unaltered for four or eight weeks, and then grow gradually to the size of a bean, never larger. They are seated in the sub-cutaneous cellular tissue, the skin over them is moveable, and adheres to the eruption the more intimately the larger it grows. After a while a number of these little swellings change to abscesses which break in the middle, discharging a thick, dark, bloody pus, and then becoming covered with a blackish scurf, beneath which they heal very soon. The ulcerative process is accompanied with loss of substance, and the cicatrices retain for a long time a hardness and a blue-red, livid color.

There are generally from fifty to one hundred papulæ which break out at various periods, so that they exist upon the skin in all their various stages. Some of them remain small, others run the course just described, all are isolated. There is no pain or fever; only if the skin remains inflamed after the falling off of the scurf, some pain is experienced.

The patients were all less than a year old; the eruption

was accompanied by other syphilides, such as scales and pustules, and more particularly flat tubercles. Most of these patients died in a state of cachexia.

Syphilis of little children has been investigated in Sweden by a special board of physicians, with the following results:

1. There is no diagnostic sign by which a cutaneous disease, pustule or ulcer, when first showing itself on a nurse or infant, could be traced to syphilis.

2. A syphilitic father may procreate a syphilitic child without infecting the mother.

3. We cannot as yet admit that a nurse's milk is alone capable of infecting an infant with syphilis.

4. Nor can a nurse be infected by an infant tainted with latent syphilis.

5. Secondary syphilis is less contagious than primary.

6. A child which is apparently healthy, when taken from a syphilitic nurse and transferred to a sound one, may infect the latter.

7. In case the life of the child should be jeopardized by feeding, a physician would not be justified by the bare suspicion of syphilis in the child or nurse, in depriving it of the nurse's milk.

8. No law should be enacted to prevent a nurse from voluntarily nursing an infant which she knows to be syphilitic.

9. In order to limit, if not to eradicate syphilis in foundling hospitals, every infant should have its own nurse.

10. If a child, whose parents are altogether unknown, is given to a nurse, she ought to be warned against the possible danger of syphilis.

11. Sores on the breasts should be attended to with great care, and, if possible, only such nurses should be engaged as have had children at the breast for some time.

12. There is no precise period when the first signs of congenital syphilis first show themselves.

13. On account of the possibility of relapses, children that have been cured of syphilis, should be carefully watched for a year longer.

In treating children for syphilis, it is above all of importance that they should not be exposed any longer to the action of the syphilitic virus. If the mother or nurse is infected with syphilis, some other healthy nurse has to be selected. Cleanliness, which is of the utmost importance in the case of full grown syphilitic patients, is so much more important in the case of little children. These little patients should be bathed every day, and kept in a uniform, somewhat more elevated temperature. If these conditions are properly observed, the homœopathic treatment of congenital syphilis will be found much more efficacious than the allopathic. In most cases, a few doses of *Mercurius sol.* will be sufficient to free the little patients of their sufferings, and to prevent all consecutive disorders. Only in very few cases it will be found necessary to resort to other remedies. If no cure should be effected by a few doses of Merc. sol., *Mercurius præcipitatus ruber.*, *Mercurius dulcis.*, or *Vivus* may be tried. If the child should improve in looks, the ulcers should heal and the little patient gain flesh, we may safely conclude that the syphilitic disease has been reached in its fundamental principles, and if some symptoms should still remain lingering in the organism, we have to treat them in accordance with the homœopathic law, "*similia similibus.*" If circumstances should render it impossible to engage another nurse, the sick mother or nurse has to be treated simultaneously with the child, and the same remedies will have to be given.

SECOND SERIES.

Non-Syphilitic Diseases of the Sexual Organs.

The number of non-syphilitic diseases of the sexual organs is likewise very great. They occur as frequently and are as injurious to the organism as the syphilitic diseases. Not only do they make terrible inroads upon both body and mind, and even destroy them entirely; they deprive man of the noblest function which God has appointed him to perform, the pro-creation of offspring, and of the sweetest delights which a man can enjoy, namely the delights of pure and true love.

A great many derangements of the sexual organs arise from depraved sensuality and from the horrible practice of self-abuse to the pernicious consequences of which upon body and mind we shall devote particular attention. But there are likewise other affections of these parts which owe their origin to either causes, abnormal, social or constitutional influences, an abnormal structure of the parts, and a variety of other more or less evident circumstances.

We will first treat of the latter class of diseases, and afterwards of those which are the natural consequences of sexual abuse, together with the most appropriate treatment for their removal.

Hydrocele.

By hydrocele we understand an effusion of serum into the tunica vaginalis testis, and into the spermatic cord. The tunica vaginalis of the testes and spermatic cord is a serous membrane which, like other serous membranes, consists of two layers between which a little serum is seated on its inner surface. This serous membrane is always moist, smooth, lubricated, owing to the serous fluid which is exhaled by the blood vessels and absorbed again by the lymphatics. If more serum is secreted than is absorbed by the lymphatics, it accumulates between the layers of the tunica vaginalis.

This excess of secretion is most frequently owing to sanguineous congestion and an inflammatory irritation of the tunica vaginalis, and sometimes developes itself quite rapidly.

Hydrocele may occur at every age, even in new-born children, but it is most frequent among the young. The most ordinary exciting causes are: constant riding on horseback, bruises, contusions, badly applied trusses, inflammations of the urethra and testicles.

The scrotum swells to the shape of a pear, generally on one side; the swelling is elastic, and if percussed simultaneously on both sides, fluctuation is perceived in it. The lower portion of the scrotum swells first; sooner or later the swelliag rises towards the inguinal ring. The size of the swelling varies, at first from the size of a pear to that of a fist. According as there is more or less serum in the tumor, it is either soft and elastic, or hard and tense, so that it might easily be confounded with sarcocele, which is very apt to happen in hydrocele of long standing where the tunica vaginalis is considerably thicker than usual.

In some cases the swelling spreads as far as the middle of the thighs and even the knees, and is distinctly seen through the pantaloons. The skin of the scrotum remains unaltered except that the blood-vessels become a little more prominent.

Hydrocele is not a painful disease, and what pain there is, is generally slight, and caused by the pulling of the spermatic cord, and the pressure upon the testicle.

The safest diagnostic is the transparency of the swelling, if, in a dark room, a light is held in front of it, and the swelling is examined from behind.

The fluid which is contained in the swelling, is generally clear, yellowish, frequently contains a number of crystals of cholestearine, smells of semen, and consists of a quantity of water, albumen, phosphates, sulphates, and muriates. Less frequently the fluid is turbid, green, brownish, or deep brown.

If the fluid is mixed up with a good deal of blood, the affection is termed *hæmatocele.*

Of itself hydrocele is not a dangerous disease. Persons may have it for years without feeling any pain. But if the swelling grows to a very large size, pains in the spermatic cord and renal region may be experienced. On account of the enormous size of the swelling, the penis becomes very short; sometimes it is entirely concealed, and sexual intercourse becomes impossible. The discharge of urine is interfered with, and the emission of semen is likewise impeded.

Hydrocele of young people, if of recent origin, may be cured by the following remedies:

Calcarea carb., Conium, Digitalis, Dulcamara, Mercurius sol., Spongia, Staphys.

[Of these remedies *Calcarea* and *Spongia* may be principally used, when there seems to be a scrofulous taint pervading the constitution, and the reproductive system is depressed, as indicated by loss of appetite, debility, emaciation, dryness of the skin.

Conium is particularly suitable when the affection can be traced to mechanical injuries, contusions, etc.

Dulcamara, when it arises from a cold, suppression of tetters, suppression of momentary or habitual sweat by exposure to a draught of air, dampness, etc.

Mercurius sol., if the patient had been troubled, when a little child, with soreness and swelling of the sexual organs, especially of the prepuce, if he is liable to feeling chilly and taking cold during damp weather, with sore throat worse during empty deglutition; if the hair is dry, falls out, the patient is troubled with sour-smelling night-sweats, costiveness, the alvine evacuations being hard, dark-colored, lumpy.

Digitalis may prove useful if there is a constant desire to pass water, or if the patient had had water in the brain when a child.]

In the case of little children we may use *Pulsatilla* and *Rhus tox.* in the commencement of the disease, and afterwards *Carbo veg., Graph., Helleb.* and *Iodine.*

[Graphites is particularly useful in such cases. *Iodine* is adapted to a general scrofulous taint, characterized by glandular swellings, emaciation. *Helleborus* when the child had had water on the brain, or dropsy after scarlet fever.]

In the case of plethoric individuals, we may have to use *Arsenic*, *China*, *Ignatia* or *Nux vomica;* (Arsenic more particularly if the glans penis is inflamed and swollen, and *Nux vomica* if the patient has a ravenous desire for meat, bowels are costive, and the patient is troubled with piles, and has an irritable disposition.) If the disease is of long standing, or very extensive, we may try *Ferrum*, *Silicea*, *Sulphur* and *Zincum*. In old people, where absorption has become impossible, tapping, or even extirpation may have to be resorted to.

Varicocele, Cirsocele.

By varicocele we mean a morbid dilatation of the veins of the spermatic cords and testicles.

The causes of this somewhat frequent disease are, in some respects anatomical, inasmuch as the veins of the spermatic cords form long sinuosities, and are so arranged that blood has overcome its own gravitation, which is rendered still more difficult by the absence of valves in the veins. Persons who are naturally disposed to varices and piles, are liable to varicocele. Beside these mechanical causes, the disease may likewise be caused by excessive sexual intercourse, and by onanism, owing to the permanently increasing congestion which these practices determine to the sexual organs. Habitual costiveness becomes a mechanical cause of this disease, in consequence of the reflux of the venous blood being impeded by the hard fæces which are lodged in the lower portion of the colon. This explains the fact why the disease occurs more frequently on the left side, where the left spermatic vein passes under the last portion of the colon. In a similar manner a tumor in and on the abdomen, or a large hernia of long standing, may produce varicocele by pressure upon the spermatic cord. Constant riding on horseback, and continual standing during work, likewise favor the development of the disease. Badly applied trusses, venous congestions of the abdomen, or of the portal system, swelling of the liver will sometimes cause the disease. A varicocele of considerable size, which involves the inguinal canal, may be mistaken for scrotal hernia. Its slow disappearance in a horizontal, and its equally slow return in an upright position constitute characteristic differences between the two diseases.

Varicocele is characterised by the following phenomena: A soft, knotty and elastic swelling extends from the scrotum to the inguinal ring; the nodosities readily disappear under pressure, but reappear again as rapidly. The scrotum hangs down relaxed; the affected side is longer; the more the disease progresses, the longer and the more relaxed becomes the scrotum. The swelling decreases in a recumbent posture, it increases after standing and walking, hence the swelling generally reaches its largest size in the evening. On pressing upon the scrotum, a sensation as of a bundle of worms is experienced. The pains are, upon the whole, not very considerable; at times dull pains in the loins and kidneys, a feeling of heaviness, malaise, drawing in the spermatic cord and testicles; shooting, colicky stitches are occasionally experienced in these regions, especially when the sexual desire is excited without an opportunity being given of gratifying it. Such shooting stitches are generally experienced when dallying with a handsome woman. The patients feel easier by supporting the scrotum with the hand. On the inner side of the thigh which is in contact with the diseased testicle, the patients generally perspire a good deal; the sweat which is generally of a corrosive character, frequently causes a troublesome eczema on the scrotum and thigh, sometimes spreading to the perinæum and anus. The affection never endangers life, but is troublesome and wears upon the spirits. At times the pains become more acute, strike to the renal region and thighs; walking is impeded. These disagreeable sensations in the sexual parts cause depression of spirits, fretfulness, and hypochondria. The patients are continually haunted by the idea of being affected by an incurable malady, are frequently driven to suicide by such thoughts.

As we have said, the disease is not dangerous to life, nor is the sexual power necessarily affected by it. Nevertheless, if the spirit should be much affected, and the disease should have attained a high degree of development, the treatment will have to be conducted with care and energy.

Lighter cases of this disease may yield to cold hip-baths, suspensaries, and to the abstaining from all influences which have a tendency to promote a congestion of blood to the parts, such as: sexual intercourse, riding on horseback, dancing, constant walking or standing, warm baths, etc. For the depression of spirits we may use: *Belladonna, Calc. carb., Caustic., Conium, Lycopod., Pulsat., Sepia, Tart. stib., Veratrum.*

Varicocele of the labia majora is of less frequent occurrence. It is less troublesome than varicocele of the scrotum, and generally yields to a few doses of *Lycopodium.*

[The medicines may be used in the following order:

Belladonna, if the patient suffers with symptoms of congestion in other parts, especially in the head, and the swelling feels hot, hard, with stitching and throbbing pains.

Calcarea carb., may be given in alternation with, or after Belladonna, especially if the sexual instinct is very much excited, the skin and hair are dry, the bowels are costive.

Lycopodium and *Sepia* may be used in the place of Calcarea, if the sexual desire is depressed and the sexual power is likewise very weak.

Pulsatilla is particularly suited to individuals of a plegmatic, melancholy disposition, and who are subject to gastric derangements, mucous diarrhœa, bad taste in the mouth, etc., in recent cases.

Aconite will be found eminently useful in raising the nervous energies of the affected part, and dispelling the engorgement of the vessels.]

Derangements of the Menstrual Functions.

Menstruation is an exclusive function of the sexual organs of the human female, and a regular recurrence of this phenomenon is of great importance to a healthful condition of her sexual powers. Derangements, irregularities or suppressions of the menstrual functions are frequently the cause of many diseases of the uterine system, and even of *sterility*.

The appearance of the menses, together with other changes in the female organism, is a sign that the sexual system of the female is maturely developed. In one climate the average appearance of the menses is about the fifteenth year, and their cessation from the forty-fifth to the fiftieth. In warm climates, among the inhabitants of the southern region, the menses both appear and and cease at an earlier period. The appearance of the menses is hastened by the woman's mode of life, her morals, the use of highly seasoned food, and premature sexual intercourse. If the menses are regular, they ought to reappear every four weeks. In a state of health, they last four days, sometimes from five to eight days. As a general rule, the menses do not flow during pregnancy and while the woman is nursing; in a very few cases, however, the menses were known to have continued during pregnancy.

This monthly discharge of blood, which is necessary to a healthy female, is subject to frequent derangements and irregularities which require an appropriate medical treatment. The menses are frequently preceded or accompanied by pains in the sacral region and abdomen, drawing in the thighs, stitches in the breasts, headache, vomiting and other nervous symptoms. During the menstrual flow the woman is generally paler than usual, tired, not disposed to work; the eyes are somewhat sunken, surrounded by blue margins. Such symptoms are of no importance, and do not require the interference of art; as soon as the menses cease, the woman's spirits become brighter, and the desire for sexual intercourse is restored.

Suppression of the menses at a period when they ought to flow with regularity, is a morbid condition of the organism, termed amenorrhœa.

This condition is characterised by a variety of troublesome symptoms. About the period when the menses ought to flow, the patients frequently complain of violent pains in the small of the back and loins, drawing and heaviness in the feet, more frequent urging to urinate, malaise in the abdomen, irritable mood, and hysteric spasms. Signs of congestion in other organs are frequently present, such as headache, vertigo, buzzing in the ears or oppression of the chest, spitting of blood, palpitation of the heart, cramps in the stomach, vomiting, etc. Even convulsions may set in; in the more favorable cases the nose bleeds. Between these periodical paroxysms, symptoms of plethora are frequently present, the patients feel heavy, weary, their sleep is uneasy. In many cases chlorotic symptoms gradually develope themselves and may even terminate in dropsy.

In amenorrhœa the menses are retained from the first; an accidental suppression of the menses after they had made their appearance, is termed menoschesis.

The menstrual suppressions may either be complete, where there is no flow at all, or only partial, with scanty discharge.

The menstrual flow may be suddenly arrested by violent emotions, such as fright, anger; exposure of the feet, chest or sexual parts to dampness, a draught of air, keen winds; immoderate dancing; leaving off a portion of the underclothes; suppression of sweat on the feet; coït during the menses; fever and other acute diseases.

Scanty menstruation occurs in chlorotic females, affected with leucorrhœa, or after considerable losses of the animal fluids, after severe diseases, puerperal fevers, or in consequence of deficient care and food. It has often been observed that women of the age of thirty or forty suddenly gain flesh, whereas, at the same time, the menses flow more scantily, and even sterility sets in. Diseases of the uterus, ovaries and vagina may induce scanty menstruation or a complete suppression of the menstrual flow.

Suppressed or scanty menstruation is generally accompanied by congestions, hœmorrhages from the nose, mouth, stomach, bowels, lungs, bladder, rectum, skin, breasts, or from existing ulcers. The nervous system is likewise affected, and we have hysteria, epilepsy, corea, catalepsy, spinal irritation, cardialgia, neuralgia, somnambulism, mental derangements, paralysis, etc. Disorganizations leading to consumption, hectic fever and dropsy may likewise set in.

In investigating the causes of menstrual suppression, we have to pay particular attention to the probable existence of pregnancy. The general phenomena, such as nausea, vomiting, nervous derangements, congestions, etc., are very much alike in both conditions; the abdomen may even bloat considerably. Some women, especially when young, and recently married, mistake the symptoms of amenorrhœa for pregnancy.

Dysmenorrhœa is another form of menstrual irregularity. It is a flow of the menses accompanied with much distress. The discharge is not suppressed, but sometimes preceded for several days; and accompanied by acute distress.

Sometimes the flow is excessively copious, and almost resembles hæmorrhage. General debility, anæmia, dropsy and sterility may arise from such a state.

For amenorrhœa the following remedies will be found most suitable:

Baryt. carb., Belladonna, Calcar. carbon., Causticum, Cocculus, Conium, Dulcam., Kali. carb., Lycop., Magnes. mur., Mercur. sol., Mezer., Natr. mur., Pulsat., Sepia, Spongia, Staphys.

For menstrual suppression we give: *Arsen. alb., Alum., Con., Coccul., Ferrum, Ignat., Graphit., Natr. mur., Nux. vom., Platin., Plumb., Opium, Sepia, Sulphur.*

In dysmenorrhœa the following medicines have proved efficacious:

Acon., Antim. crud., Aurum., Bellad., Calc. carb., Carbo.

veg., *Coccul.*, *Conium*, *China*, *Graphit.*, *Ipec.*, *Iodine*, *Magnes. carb.*, *Natrum*, *Natrum mur.*, *Nux mosch.*, *Phosphor.*, *Pulsat.*, *Stramon.*, *Sulphur*, *Veratr.*

I have derived particular benefit from the alternate use of *China* and *Nux vom.*

In menorrhagia or excessive menstruation, I have given with great success:

Acid. nitr., *Acon.*, *Arnic.*, *Arsen.*, *Bellad.*, *Chamom.*, *China*, *Crocus*, *Coccul.*, *Ferrum*, *Ignat.*, *Nux vom.*, *Platina*, *Sepia*, *Silicea*, and *Sulphur*.

[For the benefit of the reader we give the following symptomatic indications of the principal remedies in this list:

Aconite is a great remedy for menstrual suppression in consequence of fright, exposure to wet or a draught of air, with soreness all over, and particularly in the lower part of the abdomen; oppression on the chest, palpitation of the heart, headache, dizziness, buzzing in the ears; also for metrorrhagia, with burning sensation in the womb, the blood is bright-red, the flow is accompanied with chills and flushes of heat, fainting feeling, throbbing in the whole body, heaviness of the lower limbs.

Cocculus: Premature menses, with distension of the abdomen, contractive cutting in the abdomen at every movement and when drawing breath, sharp pressure as from stones in the distended abdomen when sitting or moving, painfulness of the distended abdomen as from an ulcer; amenorrhœa with abdominal spasms, flatulence, lameness, anguish, oppression of breathing, spasms in the chest, nausea with fainting sensation; painful menstruation with copious discharge of coagula and subsequent hæmorrhoids; suppression or irregularity of the menses, with uterine spasms.

Arsenicum: Painful menstruation, with lancinations from the rectum to the anus and pudendum, or from the pit of the stomach to the hypogastrium, weeping and moaning.

Ignatia: Scanty menstruation, with black blood, having a putrid odor.

Magnesia muriatica: Profuse menstruation, with pain in

the small of the back and thighs, also spasms in the ligaments of the uterus.

Nux vomica: Premature menses, more scanty than usual, also with nausea, chilliness and fainting, which is sometimes preceded by spasmodic movements in the abdomen, and followed by a sense of chilliness on rising from bed; painful menstruation, with contractive uterine spasms, a griping and digging sensation, with discharge of clots of coagulated blood.

Ipecacuanha, in metrorrhagia, with nausea, faint feeling; also, after miscarriage.

Pulsatilla, Amennorrhœa caused by a cold, with pale face, spasmodic tightness in the chest after the slightest emotion, chilliness even in summer; amenorrhœa with leucorrhœa, vertigo, throbbing headache, fulness and pressure in the stomach, drawing, aching pain in the uterus, painful micturition; painful menstruation, with cutting in the abdomen and uterus, pressure on the bladder, loss of appetite, discharge of black and viscous blood: painful menstruation, preceded and accompanied by pleuritic stitches, which are excited by moving the arms, drawing breath, and by loud talking, and laming the arm; menstruation, with thick and black blood, discharged by fits and starts.

Sepia, premature menses, with scanty flow, leucorrhœa with stitches in the uterus, and itching in the vagina.

Sulphur is indicated, for similar conditions as Sepia, especially if the menstrual blood is thick, black, and so acrid that it renders the thigh sore.

Platina will be found serviceable for excessive menstruation, with pressing from the groins to the genital organs, and spasmodic labor-like pains in the abdomen; dark blood, which is partly fluid and partly coagulated; metrorrhagia, with sexual orgasm and desire for an embrace; also, with thirst, anorexia, sensation as if a ball were moving about in the abdomen, pressing pains in the groins; also, with sensation as if the body were growing larger in every direction.

Crocus, metrorrhagia, the blood being dark and coagulated.

Sabina, metrorrhagia, with bright red arterial blood.

China, metrorrhagia, with drawing in the lower abdomen and thighs, sense of debility, bearing down pains in the womb, sallow complexion, dizziness, chilliness, stretching of the limbs.

Secale cornutum, metrorrhagia with bearing down pains, resembling labor-pains.]

There is one remedial agent which has helped me out in the most obstinate and inveterate cases of amenorrhœa, where every other means had failed. This agent is electro-magnetism, which I have found to be one of the most efficient means in many diseases of the sexual organs, and concerning which, I offer more extensive remarks at the conclusion of the chapter on the consequences of sexual excesses.

I have treated many cases of amenorrhœa, accompanied with considerable derangements of the sexual sphere, and of the organism generally. These patients had been under allopathic and hydropathic treatment, but without any success. Homœopathic treatment seemed likewise inefficient, and the application of electro-magnetism was the only means by which the menses could be brought on, sometimes after a few applications only. The organism was restored to its normal condition, the sexual desire became again active, the patients looked better, and were enabled to enjoy the exquisite delight of bringing forth healthy and strong children.

In applying the apparatus, I introduced one of the poles into the vagina, and applied the other pole to the small of the back. At first, I allowed the electric current to continue for two minutes only, and then added one minute at every sitting, until the application lasted fifteen minutes, after which the menses soon made their appearance.

On Self-Abuse.

The desire to propagate the species, is one of the most sacred instincts of the human heart. This instinct, which begins to be felt about the period of pubescence, first announces itself by a mysteriously magnetic attraction of the senses towards each other. This attractive force is sexual love, which, as it progresses, develops sexual desire. This precious gift, which is one of the first means of promoting health and cheerfulness of mind, may, on the other hand, be so abused, as to destroy the organism, and become a source of torture and misery.

The perverse genius of man, misguided by sensuality, has been led to the most pernicious abuses of the sexual appetite, and to the most revolting refinements of sexual lust.

These sexual excesses undermine health, shorten life, destroy the happiness of families, incapacitate the male from the noble office of procreating offspring, and deprive woman of her beautiful mission of bearing children.

Believing with Jean Jacques Rousseau, Montaigne, Kampe, Jean Paul and others, that a knowledge of the devastating effects of vice is calculated to excite an aversion to vicious habits, and that many may be saved from destruction, who, without this knowledge, would lose bodily strength, mental vigor and contentment, by the odious practice of self-pollution: we feel called upon to devote a chapter to this interesting subject. We will first depict the frightful effects of sexual excesses, and afterwards endeavor to explain the means by which they may either be removed or alleviated.

Sexual Excesses.

Sexual excesses are almost as ancient as the human race. Man has, at all times, and among all nations, been given to refinements of sexual lust. It seems, however, as though the ancient races had been more corrupt in this respect than the modern. All such horrible violations of nature as pederasty, sodomism, etc., are much less frequent among us than they were among the ancient Greeks, Romans, and the Orientals.

Even the bible furnishes records of the sensuality of the Asiatic and African nations. Suffice it to mention the vices of Sodom and Gomorrha, the excesses of Ruben, Juda, and of Thomar, who may be set down as the mother of prostitutes; of Potiphar, Absolom, and even of the wise Solomon who kept a harem of a thousand women.

The ancient Egyptians were celebrated for their sexual excesses. The Lesbian love, which led to the extirpation of the clitoris, a practice which is still prevalent in modern Egypt, for the purpose of arresting this abuse, emanates from this region. In our article on Lesbian love, we will be more explicit on this point. According to Herodotus, the pyramid of Cheops was constructed by the lovers of the daughter of this king, as a reward for her favors. Of the wild excesses of Cleopatra whole volumes might be filled.

The temple of Isis in Egypt was the central locality of all the excesses of the priests.

The ancient Babylonians, Medes, and Lydians were celebrated for their debauched manners, but the licentiousness of the Persian kings beats every thing that history has recorded in the shape of human immorality. The most beautiful and most fascinating girls were sent to the Persian kings from every province of their vast empire. These girls had to anoint themselves for twelve months with salves, balsams, and myrtle, before they could be admitted to the honor of sharing a nightly debauch with their master. Even their own daughters and sisters became the concubines of the Persian kings.

There was a law in Babylon which obliged every maiden in the country to expose herself to a stranger, once in her lifetime, in the temple of Venus. The women of Carthage and Tyrus had to submit to a similar prostitution, and the money which they earned by this degradation, was their wedding-present. The women of Lydia obtained their bridal gift by similar means, and the women of Armenia were not deemed fit to be married until they had been prostituted by some stranger in the temple of Diana Anaïtis. In the temple of Belus at Babylon, at Thebes in Egypt, and at Patares in Lydia, it was the gods, or rather the priests, who honored the young maiden with their favor, and there are yet devotees in Egypt, to whom women expose themselves in public, in the belief that their conduct is well-pleasing to God.

We are well acquainted with the debaucheries to which the Greeks and Romans were addicted at the period when these nations had fallen from their high estate. Who has not heard of those bacchanalia during which young girls, in a state of intoxication, and singing amorous songs, half naked and dishevelled, committed the most horrible orgies with the men disguised as satyrs and shamelessly exposed?

Sappho rendered herself famous, not only by her songs, but also by her amorous excesses, and by the Lesbian vice which she helped to spread. The prostitute and public dancer Collytto, was worshipped in Athens as a goddess, under the name of Venus popularis. She was honored by nightly orgies under the direction of her priests.

Public depravity was still worse in ancient Rome. Cæsar bargained away his virtue to Nicomedes, king of Bythinia, who was designated as "the husband of all women, and as the wife of all men." Augustus was guilty of the blackest crimes, and the poet Ovidius was banished from the court of Rome for no other reason than because he had surprised the emperor in the act of committing incest with his own daughter. Every Roman lady, married or unmarried, sought the honor of a debauch with the emperor. They had first to undress themselves, in order to have all their secret charms or defects examined, before they could be admitted to the imperial favor. Caligula, whom nature, according to Seneca's own statement, had destined to show to the world what a monster on a throne is capable of doing, committed incest with all his sisters, even in the presence of his wife, and while eating his meal. He took off the married women in the presence of their husbands, and, after having exposed them in public, used any of them he took a fancy to. His palace was a brothel, where the most horrible vices were committed. He boasted of being the king of vice, and the most infamous excesses are charged upon him and his companions.

Messaline, wife of the imbecile Claudius, surpassed every woman of her time in vile licentiousness. Juvenal says of her: "Dressed in vile clothes, she entered her chamber in a public brothel, and, under the name of Lyciska, exposed her body that had borne the magnanimous Britannicus;

she was the last to leave the house in the morning, not satiated but wearied."

Nero went even so far as to violate the person of a vestal, a crime which the superstitious Romans would not forgive their emperor Heliogabalus.

The purifying influence of christianity arrested for some centuries theses excesses, but after this period lost all power of restraining the lusts of either rich or poor, laymen or priests. Monks and nuns were as much addicted to debauchery as the Greeks and Romans had been, so that Charlemagne was obliged to issue the following edict:

"We have been informed, to our great horror, that many monks are addicted to debauchery and all sorts of vile abominations, even to unnatural sins. We forbid all such practices in the most solemn manner, and hereby make known that all monks who indulge in the gratification of such lusts, will be punished by us so severely that no christian will ever care to commit such sins again. We command our monks to cease swarming about the country, and we forbid our nuns to practice fornication and intoxication. We shall not allow them any longer to be whores, thieves, murderers and so-forth, to spend their time in debauchery and sing improper songs. Priests are herewith forbidden to haunt the taverns and market-places for the purpose of seducing mothers and daughters, etc."

This account of sexual excesses might be continued down to our time, but it is useless to dwell upon such statistics any further. The facts which we have related, are sufficient to show that such excesses have prevailed among all nations and at all ages, and have been a prolific source of the physical and moral deterioration of our race.

Among the specific forms of a depraved sexual appetite we distinguish pederasty, the Lesbian love and sodomy; these abominations are, fortunately, rarely indulged in among modern nations; but there is one vice which is universally prevalent now-a-days, and to which we shall devote a good deal of attention, it is the vice of self-abuse or onanism.

Pederasty. This vice, horrible as it is, was practised even by the most ancient people. Among the Hebrews, whole cities were addicted to it. It is believed that Sodom and Gomorrah were destroyed by fire and brimstone as a punishment for this abominable practice. In Greece pederasty was a religious art, and the most distinguished men, even Socrates, whose minds soared far above the common ideas and habits of the race, are said to have practised this vice. Greece, Syria, Egypt, and the north of Africa and Asia, are known as countries where sodomy is a native vice. Prisoners of the Egyptian musulmans, bedouins or maures, have to submit to the infamous familiarities of their captors. In all those countries of Asia where Bramah is worshipped, there exists a class of young men who make it their business to sell themselves for such horrible purposes. Among the Christian nations of modern times the vice of pederasty has become nearly extinct. In the middle ages it prevailed to a considerable extent among the Catholic priests; even Leo X and Sixtus IV. were suspected of indulging in it. Among us pederasty is a capital crime, like murder; in 1750, two pederasts were publicly burnt in Paris. In the larger capitals of Europe some refined rake may yet now and then be found anxious to buy the favors of a few handsome young reprobates who are generally unacquainted with the evil consequences of this practice, such as fistulæ, induration and ulceration of the rectum, and in whom the last whisperings of an outraged conscience are stifled by their horrible depravity.

The so-termed Lesbian love is a vice of a still more hideous and degrading nature than pederasty. If it be a horrible practice for men to gratify their lust in filthy embraces, how much more disgusting is it to see women approach each other for the purpose of quieting their wild desires by the most unnatural intimacy. It seems as though sexual depravity could scarcely reach a lower level.

This vice has derived its name from the island of Lesbos, where it was practised by the celebrated poetess Sappho. In ancient Rome, it was likewise common; and women who indulged in it, were called by the Romans "Tribades."

Previous to the first French revolution, there existed a society of women in Paris, who numbered some of the first ladies of the city among their number, and who made it their business to practice this vice in common. As if to add mockery to their infamy, they termed themselves the society of the "vestals."

Sodomy was originally practiced by shepherds, who resorted to this mode of gratifying their sexual passion with beasts, for want of more natural opportunities. Even at this day, sodomy is still practiced in Sicily, with goats. According to Blumenbach, the women of Guinea have intercourse with monkeys, and the Persians resort to she-asses as a cure for coxalgia.

Self-Abuse, and its Consequences.

Onanism, or self-abuse, is a most pernicious vice, and a deplorable substitute for a natural gratification of the sexual passion.

According to the bible this vice was first practiced by Onan, from whom it is named; but the Greeks and Romans attribute it to the artful Mercury, who invented it for the benefit of Pan, who had lost his mistress, the beautiful Echo.

It is an unfortunate fact that this vice can be traced to the remotest antiquity, and that it has been practiced by the lowest as well as by the highest classes of society. It is a most unnatural vice, resulting in extinction of the conjugal faculty, demoralization, and weakness of the sexual powers.

The effects of this vice are the more pernicious the sooner it is practiced. In our generation it is known even to tender childhood. Thousands are initiated in such practices by servants and nurses. In public and private schools it is universally prevalent. How important it is, therefore, for parents and teachers, to watch the private conduct of their pupils.

The consequences of this vice differ more or less according to the age and sex of the patient.

Previous to the age of pubescence, the effects in both sexes are pretty nearly alike: momentary excitement, followed by depression of spirits, and finally by a more or less complete derangement of the nervous functions.

The following is a tolerably accurate picture of the gradual effects of this vice: After having indulged in this practice for a time, repeating it more and more frequently until it becomes a daily habit, the child, without being otherwise sick, loses its bright complexion, which becomes pale, with a greenish tint, especially around the eyes, which are sunken, surrounded by blue margins; the lips lose their vermillion hue. Careful observation reveals to us other important signs of the alteration of the child's health. The mind is indolent, the child sits with the head inclined forward, staring as if absorbed in deep thoughts, without, however, looking at any thing, and started by a sudden question. If told to do a thing, the child rises slowly from its seat, and all its motions are slow and heavy. It is averse to play, which it loved formerly, prefers sitting quiet and alone, becomes obstinate, peevish, irritable, and cannot bear the least joke. Children who are addicted to such habits, like to be in solitary places, where they can indulge their vicious propensities; they like to sleep late in the morning, and nevertheless feel unrefreshed and heavy on getting up. Gradually every function, especially digestion, suffers more or less. The tongue and teeth are covered with phlegm, the least nourishment causes distress, colic, oppression, flatulence. The child grows thin, and the mental faculties are weakened. The power of comprehension is diminished, the child is dull and taciturn, though unconsciously so. Such consequences may continue for years, to the end of life, even though the practice of this vice had long been abandoned, and everything had been done to restore the patient's health. If some kind of sickness should set in at this time, it is generally very severe; the least fever is apt to assume a typhoid form, and the exhausted body speedily succumbs to the ravages of disease.

Sadly does the young life perish even before it had begun to bud, as a young plant withers away at whose root a worm had been gnawing. All the cares of sorrowing parents are fruitless, the sources of their highest terrestrial happiness are drained, and the state is deprived of useful and healthy citizens.

From this short but true picture we may infer that there is no more degrading bondage than the bondage of one's own lusts. The imagination is enkindled by an impure fire. It is in vain that the patient tries to resist the power of habitual vice; it torments him in his dreams, and in his waking hours. And, instead of enjoyment, it gives him disappointment and misery. Self-abuse is the most certain road to the grave. It not only destroys the body, but likewise undermines the peace of the soul; the destruction is not accomplished all at once; slowly, but most certainly, the onanist instils a poison into his frame that will inevitably lead to death.

If this vicious habit is continued beyond the age of pubescence, the fountain of health is drained forever. The mind is weakened, the memory gone, the ideas become confused, and the patients frequently are seized with mania; they are constantly restless, tormented by anguish and remorse, and driven to tears; they are subject to frequent attacks of vertigo; their senses, especially sight and hearing, are weakened; their sleep, provided it has not entirely left them, is interrupted by uneasy dreams. The body is exhausted, its growth is checked, the patients are tormented by violent pain, such as headache, pains in the chest, pressure at the stomach, colic; all complain of an indescribable lassitude in the limbs. The face is covered with itching pimples, pustules on the nose, chest, thighs. The sexual organs suffer a good deal; some lose all power of erection; others lose their semen from the least excitement, or even at stool, while bearing down. Others, again, are afflicted with a constant flow of semen, termed spermatorrhœa. Robust persons are sometimes troubled with very painful erections. Some lose their urine involuntarily, others are attacked with a most painful retention of urine, or with violent burning at urinating. Many are attacked with swellings of the testicles, pains in the penis and spermatic cord. Most of these unfortunates are impotent, either because they are no longer capable of erections, or because the semen has lost all its vivifying properties. The functional derangements caused in other organs, will be mentioned more particularly in the sequel.

In women the consequences of onanism are somewhat different from what they are in men. The object of this vicious habit is the same in boys as well as in girls, viz.: sexual excitement. There is this difference, that girls do not weaken themselves by the loss of the spermatic fluid, but by the excessive exaltation of the nervous system. Nervous prostration is therefore the first effect of onanism in young females, and is characterized by headache, depression of spirits, obstinacy, sadness, indifference to worldly pleasures, and finally, melancholy and other forms of mental derangement. The senses become duller, especially the eyes, which are red and dim, with a staring look.

In the hospitals and lunatic asylums, there is a larger number of females than males, under treatment for onanism. This is an additional proof, that in the female, the mind and nervous system are principally affected by onanism.

This nervous derangement soon leads to a derangement of the digestive system. The patients grow thin. All sorts of spasmodic symptoms develope themselves, such as spasms, cardialgia, chorea, epilepsy, catalepsy, convulsions, etc. All the former charms of the young woman leave her, her face looks sallow and thin, the skin is rough, dry, cracked, covered with freckles and pimples; the eyes look dim, the lips are pale and bluish, the teeth decay. A copious mucus is discharged from the vagina, corroding the thighs, groins, and perinæum, and causing a most distressing hysteria. The internal organs become diseased, indurations and cancer of the womb develope themselves, and the patients either die of some such disease, or else pine away from debility.

Nevertheless, howsoever horrid the consequences of onanism seem, they may be prevented or removed by appropriate and timely treatment. By and bye we shall explain in detail, the means which we employ for this purpose. We will first advert to the pernicious consequences of excessive sexual intercourse, which are indeed less ruinous than the effects of onanism, but are likewise destructive of health.

My readers will naturally inquire, *At what age, and how often, is it proper to indulge, without injuring one's health?*

It is not very easy to answer this question, but we will nevertheless attempt it.

As regards age, it is undeniable that sexual intercourse ought not to be indulged in before the organism is fully developed, or the period of pubescence has been reached.

This may depend upon climate, geographical position, mode of life, food, race, temperament. All these causes may either hasten or retard the period of pubescence.

In the countries between the tropics, females attain their maturity much sooner than they do in the frigid or temperate zones. Some are known to have borne children at the age of 13 or 14, and at the age of 30 the menstrual functions cease. In the countries of the temperate zones, pubescence is reached by females at the age of 14, and by males at the age of 17 or 18. A few more years are required to enable them to reproduce their species.

In former times all premature marriages were forbidden by law. Lycurgus forbade men to marry before the age of 37, and women before the age of 17. According to Xenophon and Plutarch these laws were enacted for the purpose of raising a vigorous race. Aristotle required the husband to be 20 years older than his wife, in order that their fecundating powers might cease at the same period. Among the old Germans no man was allowed to have intercourse with a woman before he was 20 years old. It is to this abstinence that Julius Cæser attributes the strength and large size of these people.

Premature marriages have a pernicious influence upon the public health. The young people ruin themselves by untimely intercourse, which is moreover carried on to excess, in consequence of the passions being uncontrolled by reason. The children springing from such premature marriages, may be fitly compared to hot-house plants, and lack inherent strength and vigor. It may be laid down as a tolerably certain rule, that the male body is not fully developed before the 20th or 25th year. Previous to this period, the semen is not secreted in sufficient quantity, is not sufficiently vivifying to generate healthy life, and the children born of such imperfect parents, are weak, sickly, and scarcely ever attain the fulness of strength and growth.

If, in premature marriages, the man generally suffers more than the woman, it is probably because the mother's weakness is entailed on the fœtus.

On the other hand, if premature marriages are extremely hurtful and dangerous, an excessive delay in marrying may likewise become injurious to health. Marriages between persons of disproportionate ages are likewise attended with great inconveniences. The propagating faculty of one party may still exist, whilst it had become extinct in the other. Sterility, in such cases, is simply accidental. Young women may not bear children to enfeebled old husbands, whereas husbands of corresponding ages and sexual powers, will very speedily gratify the fervent desires of their hearts, to lavish a mother's cares upon a tenderly-beloved infant. An inevitable consequence of marriages between persons of disproportionate ages, is the physical weakness of the children. It has also been observed that the skin of young women who marry old men, becomes loose and withered, and breaks out in herpetic eruptions.

As regards the second question: *How often is it proper to indulge without injury to health?* it is equally difficult to return a general answer; for this depends, likewise, upon a variety of circumstances, race, age, temperament, and individual idiosyncrasies. History tells extraordinary feats of some men in this respect. Hercules is said to have impregnated fifty girls in one night. The Emperor Proculus boasted of having impregnated a hundred Sarmatian maidens in a fortnight.

Phares relates of a Moorish prince, that he had intercourse with forty women in three days. A woman requested protection of the king of Arragon against the passion of her husband, who used her ten times every night. The king confined him, under penalty of death, to six times a day. A mountaineer of the eastern slope of the Pyrenees, married eleven women in the space of fifteen years. He used them so often and vehemently, that all these women died of severe uterine affections. He was forbidden to marry the twelfth time.

Such extreme cases are rare. As a general rule, men would be ruined by such excesses. Physicians and physiologists of all ages, agree in opinion, that the loss of one ounce of semen is more debilitating than the loss of forty ounces of blood. Hippocrates tells us that the male semen is composed of all the fluids of the body, and is the most precious constituent of the human organization. By losing semen, man loses vital spirit. It is not to be wondered, therefore, that the excessive loss of semen enervates the body. It takes a long time for the organism to repair the loss of the seminal fluid. Twenty-four hours after a seminal discharge, the seminal vesicles are again full, but it takes a few additional days, to impart to this semen vivifying properties of a healthy nature.

Pythagoras terms the semen the flower of the blood; his disciple, Alcmeon, considered the semen a portion of the brain; Epicurus looked upon semen as a portion of the soul and body, and exhorted his disciples to take good care of this fluid, in order to preserve both their bodies and their souls.

All this shows that the most distinguished philosophers have, at all times, looked upon the male semen as the most precious secretion of the blood, and have cautioned against the wasteful use of this fluid, as something ruinous to the mind as well as the body.

As a general rule concerning the frequency of sexual intercourse, we may adopt the maxim of Luther, that "twice a week, or one hundred and four times a year, hurts neither me nor thee." Celsus says: "Coït should neither be practiced to excess, nor should it be entirely avoided. If moderately enjoyed, it stimulates and invigorates the body; excessive intercourse, on the contrary, destroys the body. Excess depends not upon the frequency, but upon the quality of the act, upon the age and temperament of the parties. Coït will not be hurtful, if it be not succeeded either by lassitude or pain."

This rule is likewise applicable to women, although women are less exhausted by intercourse than men, and preserve their strength better.

Daily experience shows that a man will ruin himself by excessive coït, whereas we see prostitutes getting fat in spite of their dissolute life. History, even, has preserved the names of women who had carried their licentious habits to the highest degree without their health being visibly affected by this libertinage. Quartilla, a Roman woman, boasted of not remembering having ever been a virgin, and of requiring the use of a man at least thirty times a day. Lysisca stood the embraces of fifty robust men in succession. Cleopatra entered in disguise the brothels of Rome, and triumphed by twenty-five times over the bravest prostitutes. In one night Messalina used one hundred and sixty men, without being satiated. Bertrand Rival relates that during the first French revolution, a beautiful and modest girl was ravished by twenty-eight hussars, and that the only bad effects of this violence, were a slight irritation of the vagina, and a few scratches, which soon healed again. On another occasion, a prostitute accommodated thirty soldiers without inconvenience. Under Theodorus' reign, a woman killed twenty-two men by sexual excesses. A physician of Paris relates the case of a woman of forty years old, who had used a man ten times a day for the last twenty-two years, and who still enjoyed good health.

Women frequently complain that their husbands do not satisfy them, but men are seldom heard to complain of their wives.

Such cases, however, are exceptions, and even these exceptions finally lead to important derangements. The constant irritation of the sexual parts finally relaxes the rectum so that it loses all contractile power; an incurable diarrhœa sets in, and the dilapidated body perishes. Excessive coït prevents conception, and leads to uterine diseases.

We will now devote a few paragraphs to the so-called aphrodisiacs, and show how far they may be safely used, and which of them have to be avoided. In spite of the warning of physicians, numbers allow themselves to be entrapped by such nostra, and to ruin themselves by the use of them.

Among the means which excite the sexual instinct without injuring health, we distinguish in the first place the influence of a pure and refined woman, and secondly, electro-magnetism. He whose nerves are not stimulated by the neighborhood of a charming woman, or by the electro-magnetic current, will likewise remain dull under the influence of spices, pills, and potions, or these things will at most produce only a momentary effect, to the great prejudice of the organism. To these means may be added vivid descriptions of the sensual delights of love, erotic songs, or pictures embodying love-scenes. In the chapter on "impotence," we shall allude with more minuteness to the use of electro-magnetism. Some vegetable preparations were likewise supposed to be endowed with aphrodisiac properties. This applies more particularly to the cryptogami, or the so-termed akotyledones of modern botanists. Gourmands know very well that truffles, mushrooms, ragoûts, etc., are not eaten alone because they tickle the palate.

Linnæus relates that a variety of the orchideas (a species of plants to which Dioscorides already attributed exciting properties) stimulates the sexual instinct of the bulls of Dalecaria. Fishes, oysters, crabs, eggs, celery, parsley, asparagus, mustard, vanilla, milk, figs, etc., are likewise supposed to be endowed with aphrodisiac properties.

The inhabitants of the Orient excite their sexual passions by opium, the use of which we would advise our readers, as little as the momentary suspension to which some Englishmen are said to resort for the purpose of enjoying the pleasurable excitement of the sexual organs which this suspension is supposed to procure. It has happened that such voluptuous sensualists were left to perish, the attendants forgetting to cut them down.

Almost all nations, but particularly the Orientals, have their peculiar aphrodisiaca, which shows that the sexual passions are highly esteemed everywhere. We repeat, however, that all such artificial excitements of the sexual organ are extremely injurious to the organism. The bangi of the Indians, and the maslac of the Turks, are said to be made of a species of hemp. If the Indians wish to enjoy voluptuous dreams, they take, previous to retiring, a potion composed of bangi, areca-nuts, ambra and musk. To excite the sexual desire, the Chinese use a root which they term ginseng, and which is more valuable than silver. The wine of ginseng has been introduced in Europe, but it does not seem to produce any great results, and may perhaps be made of a root, which is not the genuine ginseng. For similar purposes the Chinese employ a mollusk, termed holothuria, or biches de mer in France, which is found principally on the Charlotte islands and on other islands of the South Sea. This mollusk is dried and smoked, and brings a high price in China.

Beside ambra and musk, the animal kingdom gives us other excitants of the sexual organs, which are, however, dangerous to health and even to life. One of the principal ingredients of the so-called *diablotins* which are used in Italy and France, is Cantharides, or the Spanish fly. These *bonbons*, the name of which is significant of their abominable nature, were not only used by enervated rakes for the purpose of enjoying once more the delights of the sexual passions, but they were given to young girls who were intended as their victims, and whose seduction was more easily accomplished after their passions had been excited by such artificial means.

These diablotins were introduced at the courts of Henry III. and Charles IX., by the notorious Catharine of Medicis.

The bonbons which were used by Cardinal Richelieu in his latter days, and which became fashionable at the court of Louis XV., appear to have derived their principal effect from cantharides. The premature death of the celebrated poet Lucretius, is attributed by his biographers, to a stimulant which was given to him by his mistress Lucilia. The celebrated physician Ambrosius Paré, relates the case of a man who died of hœmorrhage caused by a powder of cantharides which was administered to him by his lady-love. A similar death happened to an old priest who took a small dose of cantharides to rouse the extinct sexual power. The deleterious effects of this drug may be inferred from the following sad occurrence: A young rake took it into his head to excite the sexual lust of two old male and female servants in the family, and for this purpose he administered to them secretly some tincture of cantharides. That same evening both servants were seized with such a wild desire that dangerous hæmorrhages ensued, of which the female servant suffered for a long time after.

Narcotic poisons, such as opium and stramonium, are likewise very dangerous and equally deleterious in their effects upon the organism. Boerhaave relates the following case:—An amorous old fool had won the affections of a young girl. In order to excite her passion and enjoy her charms, he administered to her, after a copious repast, a powder of stramonium in a cup of coffee. The girl became intoxicated, her eyes sparkled with love, her face was flushed, she sang amorous doggerel, lost all self-control, manifested an irresistible desire for sexual intercourse, took off her clothes, stared at her old Adonis, finally trembled while desirous of giving herself up to him, grated her teeth, and went into spasms. The enamored old wretch went for a physician, who restored her to health. After taking her coffee, she had lost all consciousness of what happened afterwards.

The so-termed philtra, elixirs of love, played an important part among the ancients. This name was given to certain potions which were supposed to be endowed with the power of either exciting or destroying love in an individual. But even in modern times there are superstitious people who believe that a person's love may be won and retained by some charmed potion. In Italy this faith is still prevalent among a great many. The witty, but rather superstitious traveller, William Müller, relates, in reference to this subject:

"The rendezvous of the Roman witches, of whom there are a great many among the young and old women of the city, is the ancient forum, now-a-days called campo-vecchio. There they meet in the night, the largest and most solemn meeting taking place in the night of St. John, when they appear in the form of black cats with fiery eyes. This transformation is effected by means of some mysterious ointment the principal ingredient of which is said to be the root of pimpinella, and which is rubbed upon the whole body. Who is not reminded by these witches of the Thessalian sorceresses? These witches make brews which either excite love or hatred, exorcise absent persons by means of magic formulas, and raise storms. Philtra were originally made in Naples. During my short stay, I saw several emaciated young men who were supposed by the people of the city, to have been brought to this condition by elixirs of love. People are, therefore, very careful not to give away their hair, because it is believed that the spell of love is fond of adhering to the hair. It is supposed that in Rome the people are more safe. During the carnival the bonbons which are thrown to one by masked persons, are generally avoided; strangers are warned against accepting them. Female masks frequently exclaim to the passer by: "Eat the bonbon, do not be afraid, you are not handsome enough to make yourself uneasy about any thing."

Although it is undeniable that these various influences tend, by their narcotic or exciting virtues, to lull the victim to sleep, or to excite the sexual passions, and facilitate the nefarious scheme of the seducer: there are, on the other hand, natural agents which exalt the sexual powers without injuring the body. We know, for instance, that the sexual instinct of cats is very much excited by valeriana, or by the nepeta cataria of Linnæus. Birds that are fed on fœnu Græcum, buckwheat, and other kinds of seed, become very much excited; even carps become heated by rubbing musk on their posterior parts.

It is well known that the exhalations of animals are influenced by the sexual act, and it was therefore believed by the ancients that such exhalations, being so intimately related to the sexual functions, must likewise exercise a powerful influence on man; the mucus which is secreted from the vagina of the mare during the act, and which was termed by them hippomanes, was supposed to be an important agent. There are other animal secretions which likewise stimulate the sexual power, for instance: castoreum, ambra, zibeth, musk. Ancient physicians used to mix all these things in their elixirs, and even corresponding human secretions were added.

Diseases arising from an excessive development of the Sexual Instinct, whether induced by artificial or natural means.

I. Satyriasis.

This disease is peculiar to men only, and is much less frequent in our climate than nymphomania, which is peculiar to females, and is characterized by similar symptoms.

The causes why this disease occurs less frequently among men than among women, are various. Man enjoys more freedom than woman to gratify his sexual passion, he leads a more active life, gets more tired by his labor, whereas woman, especially in the higher walks of society, seems to live almost exclusively for the purpose of indulging in sensations of every kind.

Satyriasis is characterized by the following phenomena: permanent erection, an excessive, insatiable desire for sexual intercourse, which sometimes increases to a perfect frenzy. The outbreak of the disease is generally preceded by frequent, passing erections, which occur either spontaneously or at the sight of women. The imagination is continually tormented by lascivious images; sleep is disturbed by dreams, and by frequent seminal emissions; the desire for sexual intercourse is constantly increasing, and is gratified indiscriminately in every shape and manner. The patient is attacked with an acute fever, the face looks fiery, the glistening eyes protrude from their sockets, the mouth foams, the patient complains of a burning thirst, becomes delirious, raves about the most horribly lascivious things, and has to be prevented by force from indulging in the most abominable self-gratifications. If the patient is not speedily relieved by adequate treatment, the sexual organs become inflamed, gangrenous, and death terminates his horrible sufferings.

This disease may be caused by excessive sexual intercourse, onanism, aphrodisiac medicines, especially cantharides, frequent reading of lascivious novels, irritations of the skin by eruptions, flaggellations, excessive abstemiousness. In respect to this last point, the history of pastor Blanchet, narrated by himself, is very remarkable. Firmly struggling against the sexual passions from his boyhood, he fled the other sex. But being of a robust constitution, he was attacked with satyriasis at the age of 32 years, and was almost driven to frenzy. His health was restored by the moderate enjoyment of the sexual passion.

The treatment should not only be medicinal, but the mind of the patient has likewise to be acted upon by adequate treatment. The imagination of the patient should be quieted by cautiously and gradually presenting to it images of female purity and loveliness, and the mind should be occupied by mechanical exercises or easy intellectual labor; mechanical labor has likewise to be resorted to. Other means of cure are: cold baths, douches, cold hip-baths several times a day, moderate and cooling diet and drinks, sleeping on hard mattresses.

Among the remedies which are useful in this disease, and which have to be chosen with reference to the bodily as well as to the moral symptoms, we distinguish the following:

Agaricus, Agnus castus, Anacardium, Antimonium cru-

dum, *Arnica*, *Asafœtida*, *Asparagus*, *Aurum*, *Baryta carbon.*, *Calcar. carbon.*, *Camphora*, *Cannabis*, *Cantharides*, *Causticum*, *Chin. mur.*, *Crocus*, *Digitalis*, *Ginseng*, *Graphites*, *Ignat.*, *Kali carbon.*, *Moschus*, *Nitric acid.*, *Phosphorus*, *Stramonium.*

(The principal remedies among this list are,

Asparagus, for sexual excitement, burning in the urethra, the urine being covered with a white pellicle, and depositing a fatty substance on the sides of the vessel.

Cantharides: Frantic sexual desire, with priapism and excessive pains.

Digitalis: Sexual excitement, with frequent and painful erections at night and in the day-time.

Ginseng: Sexual desires, with erections, lascivious dreams.

Moschus: Violent sexual desire, also with nausea and vomiting after an embrace.

These are the only agents that seem to have any positive curative virtues in this disease, and they will doubtless cure every case that admits of being cured.)

II. Nymphomania.

This disease arises from the same causes as satyriasis; such as: onanism, sexual excesses, etc.; if neglected, it generally terminates in craziness. The disease is characterized by a violent desire for sexual intercourse; such patients lose all sense of shame, expose themselves to others, and utter the vilest and most obscene speeches.

This disease occurs most frequently at the period of pubescence. Women endowed with an exquisite nervous sensitiveness, or robust women, with a profuse crop of dark hair, dark and lively eyes, expressive and animated features, and well-developed sexual organs, such as: a hard and round bosom, well-marked hips, tall stature, a large pudendum, a prominent clitoris, are particularly predisposed for this disease. All these attributes may, however, be wanting, and nymphomania may nevertheless break out. In such cases the disease is generally caused by some eruption near the sexual organs, worms, ascarides in the vagina, etc.

If nymphomania is fully developed, it presents a group of most repulsive phenomena. Such women assail every man who comes near them, supplicate and excite him by the most shameless requests to gratify their passions. Every new gratification increases the desire. If men are not at hand to quiet them, they resort to the most horrible means of self-gratification, which it is impossible to describe without shuddering.

The treatment of this disease implies the regulation of the diet and moral impressions of the patient. Exercise, employment, travelling, cold baths, cold douches, early rising from bed, and absence of all confinement in a room, are indispensable means of cure. The reason of the patients has likewise to be appealed to. Among the internal remedies, *Platina* seems to have produced the best results. A successful treatment, however, requires that all the symptoms which do not directly bear upon the sexual sphere, should be carefully investigated. If the patients' eyes look glassy, their faces are flushed, *Belladonna* and *Conium* are indicated. In other cases we may employ *Aconite*, *Arsen.*, *Canthar.*, *Ferrum*, *Hyoscyam.*, *Ignat.*, *Phosphor.*, *Pulsat.*, *Sabina*, *Sepia*, *Silicea*, *Stramonium*, *Sulphur*, and *Veratrum album*.

[*Aconite* is an admirable remedy for nymphomania characterized by a violent and distressing titillating sensation in the clitoris.

Cantharis: burning in the pudendum, violent itching in the vagina, pressing towards the genital organs.

Hyoscyamus: nymphomania accompanied with delirium, loss of all shame, desire to expose one's self.

Ignatia: nymphomania, with deep melancholy.

Pulsatilla: nymphomania with suppression of the menses, heat and weight in the pudendum.

Platina: excessive titillation in the uterus.]

III. Involuntary Seminal Emissions. Spermatorrhœa.

Spermatorrhœa is one of the most frequent, obstinate, and disastrous consequences of sexual excesses, particularly of long-continued onanism. This weakness, which only exists in the case of man, poisons every pleasure, and frequently drives man to craziness and suicide. The disease is quite frequent now-a-days, but the phenomena which characterize it, are generally attributed to some derangement of a cardinal portion of the nervous system, particularly the spinal marrow, although such nervous derangements are generally secondary, sympathetic affections. Thanks to the microscope and to a correct analysis of the urine, we find it easy to diagnose the disease; and we are likewise enabled, by the progress of science, to cure it, provided the patient is willing to obey the instructions of his physician.

Spermatorrhœa is the most frequent cause of impotence, concerning which Hippocrates already remarks: "This disease frequently occurs among the recently-married, and in consequence of sexual excesses; there is no fever, the appetite remains good, but the strength vanishes, and the patients grow thin. They complain of formication from the head down the spine; semen is lost with the urine, and at stool, also during sleep, with or without dreams, or while riding on horseback, or during a walk. The patients become impotent, debilitated, the head feels heavy, and they experience a buzzing in the head. If fever supervenes, the patients die of consumption, etc.

The semen may escape in a threefold manner:

1. During stool, at the termination of an emission of urine, during sudden motions, conversation with females, or while reading lascivious novels or songs.

2. At night, while dreaming, with or without any particular sensations, frequently only towards morning, when the bladder and rectum are full; in the more advanced stages of the disease the semen escapes while lying on the back, or sleeping on the sofa. Generally the patients wake during the

emission, at other times the loss is perceived only by the stains on the linen.

3. The semen is mixed up with the urine; there is no erection, nor any peculiar sensation of pleasure. This is spermatorrhœa in the genuine sense of the term. This is the most dangerous form of spermatorrhœa, because it is not perceived until it has developed its disastrous consequences in the organism. In some cases several of these various forms of spermatorrhœa co-exist in the same individual; but as a general rule, only one form exists at a time; some lose the semen with the urine without having ever been troubled with emissions; others lose semen during an exertion, but never with the urine; generally, however, the influence upon the organism is the same in these various cases.

Besides the above-mentioned causes of this disease, sexual excesses of various kinds, there are still other causes which it is important to investigate in order to regulate the treatment accordingly.

Sometimes the disease arises from the joint action of several causes, in which case it is difficult to ascertain the leading one. Pathologically, the phenomena of this disease may be divided into two chief categories: an irritation of the lower portion of the spinal marrow, and secondly, an irritation and chronic inflammation of the ejaculatory canals, and seminal vesicles. As regards the special causes, the following may be looked upon as the principal ones which are instrumental in producing this disease:

1. *Gonorrhœa*, especially chronic gonorrhœa. This is generally located in the posterior portion of the urethra, where the seminal ducts terminate. Hence the necessity of removing, as soon as possible, even the lighter forms of this disease.

2. *Irritating injections in the urethra.* These injections, if used to excess, or at improper periods, or if too acrid, frequently cause the inflammation of the mucous membrane to extend to the posterior portion of the urethra.

3. *Strictures of the urethra.* Behind the stricture the

urethra generally enlarges, the mucous membrane is irritated by the urine which collects in the enlarged portion, an increased quantity of mucus is secreted, and the inflammation generally spreads to the more deep-seated portions of the urethra. While endeavoring to expel the urine, the orifices of the seminal ducts become relaxed, and the involuntary discharge of semen is facilitated thereby.

4. *Morbid conditions of the rectum*, such as obstinate constipation, piles, painful fistulæ of the anus, tumors, diarrhœa. Some of these conditions act mechanically in consequence of the effort which is required during stool; others, like the piles, by communicating the irritation to the seminal vesicles.

5. *Onanism.* This is undoubtedly the most frequent cause of spermatorrhœa. This disastrous habit induces a constant irritation of the sexual organs, a more frequent and more copious determination of blood to these parts, which is alone sufficient to cause a loss of semen. After such an irritation has lasted for a time, the internal sexual parts become weaker, relaxed, particularly the orifices of the seminal ducts, in consequence of which the seminal fluid escapes more easily.

6. *Sexual excesses with women.*—These injurious consequences are of a three-fold kind: First, an increased secretion of semen in consequence of the frequent irritation of the sexual parts; *secondly*, relaxation of the whole body, and particularly of the sexual organs; thirdly, irritation and even chronic inflammation of the seminal vesicles and the ejaculatory ducts, which may be inferred from the suddenness with which the semen is discharged, and from the pain by which the discharge is accompanied. The bad effect is still increased by retaining the semen as long as possible, either for the purpose of perpetuating the pleasurable excitement, or from some other cause. By this means the vesicles and the ducts become distended, and the orifices of the ducts lose their tone and elasticity.

7. *Frequent excitation of the sexual instinct*, without subsequent natural gratification, either by lascivious books, or by intimacies with females, except sexual intercourse. In

consequence of this excitement, there is a considerable rush of blood to the sexual parts, the penis swells, becomes erect, and such erections last much longer than during an embrace; a viscous transparent fluid, the prostatic fluid, or even real semen, is discharged from the urethra; a violent throbbing sensation is experienced in the perinæal region, the face becomes flushed, the heart beats more violently, and a frequent repetition of such fruitless intimacies, brings on formication and shooting stitches in the back. The immediate consequence of this exaltation is a relaxation of the seminal vesicles, and of the orifices of the seminal ducts, which are endowed with a similar but weaker power as the sphincter muscles of other orifices of excretory ducts.

8. *Abstemiousness.* Excessive abstemiousness may likewise be attended with involuntary seminal losses. With many persons, abstemiousness is no virtue, because they are not tempted by enjoyment, and there is no virtue without temptation. There are men who practice abstemiousness from religious motives, at the expense of their health. In a full-grown young man, especially if he lives well, the testicles constantly secrete semen which ought to be discharged from time to time, proportionally to its quantity and the rapidity with which it is secreted. If this discharge is not effected by coït, the excess is got rid of by involuntary nocturnal emissions, the frequency of which is proportionate to the quantity of semen secreted. As long as these nocturnal emissions take place moderately, they afford a feeling of ease rather than otherwise. But it frequently happens that these emissions take place every night, especially if the patient had been given to excessive intercourse previous to becoming abstemious.

9. *Diseases of the cerebellum and the spinal marrow.* We know by physiological experimentation that the cerebellum and the medulla oblongata are in close relation to the sexual organs. It has been noticed that a disorganization of the cerebellum impairs the sexual functions, and that a complete atrophy of the cerebellum is succeeded by their complete

extinction. Gall already directed attention to the fact that the cerebellum is the seat of the sexual power. In his craniology we find a number of cases going to show that certain diseases of the brain, such as: inflammation, tumors, mechanical injuries inflicted by a blow, concussion, etc., cause a violent excitement of the sexual passion, and consequent seminal emissions.

Various diseases of the spinal marrow are still more frequent causes of spermatorrhœa, because a flow of semen is a standing symptom of many such spinal irritations, and consequently increases the debility. In these diseases the sexual organs are deprived of the normal nervous influence which they require for the healthy exercise of their functions. Sometimes the semen is secreted in too large a quantity, but too thin and not sufficiently vivifying. The seminal vesicles are overfilled; the excretory ducts become relaxed, as is the case with the sphincter vesicæ under similar circumstances; the testicles hang down relaxed; shooting stitches are experienced in the spermatic cord; the erections are either imperfect or entirely wanting, and an unavoidable consequence of this condition is impotence, tabes dorsalis, etc., of which mention will be made hereafter.

10. *Excessive length of the prepuce*, and consequent phymosis, may likewise lead to involuntary emissions, caused by inflammation of the surface of the glans, sensitiveness of the glans, copious accumulation of smegma behind the corona glandis. This sensation spreads from the glans to the inner parts, and causes involuntary emissions. Such emissions are, however, easily arrested.

11. In a number of cases an involuntary loss of semen is hereditary. We know this from actual observation.

12. Excessive use of tea and coffee likewise causes seminal losses. It is true that both tea and coffee act powerfully upon the kidneys, but their injurious effect upon the sexual organs is not yet proven, although a number of persons who were afflicted with seminal losses, have said that their trouble became much worse after the use of coffee or tea.

13. *Aphrodisiaca, cantharides, violent cathartics, warm and irritating injections,* cause an increased flow of blood to the pelvic organs and sexual parts, and consequently an irritation of the seminal vesicles leading to seminal losses. The injurious effects of such agents have been described before, and our readers are referred to those pages.

14. In a former paragraph we alluded to *intestinal worms,* and stated that they were capable of irritating the sexual organs. It is especially ascarides which are capable of exciting spermatorrhœa, by causing a violent irritation of the internal sexual organs, in consequence of their irritating action upon the nervous system generally. This circumstance deserves particular notice from the fact that the presence of such worms is easily overlooked; whereas, if the cause were properly noticed, its removal could easily be effected.

15. Besides the above-mentioned causes, there are others which may give rise to spermatorrhœa, such as *riding on horseback,* in consequence of the continued pressure and shaking of the genital organs; *a sedentary mode of life* which is apt to induce constipation and an increased warmth of the abdominal organs by congestions of the portal system, and lastly various *idiosyncrasies* which it is not always possible to account for upon physiological principles. There are cases where patients had not felt well for a time and afterwards were suddenly attacked with copious nocturnal emissions, without any of the causes which we have enumerated, being present. I have known a case where a man who had entered a house of dubious character, was suddenly seized with a copious loss of semen without erection, and without the least thrill, merely from fright. Many persons are attacked with seminal losses on looking down from a height, or while fancying they are lying on the border of a precipice, or while balancing themselves on a swing.

As regards the phenomena which generally accompany spermatorrhœa, we have to consider in the first place whether the seminal losses take place in the day-time or at night.

Nocturnal emissions are at first accompanied by lascivious dreams, erections and pleasurable sensations. As the trouble increases these sensations grow less, and the loss of semen is only revealed by the moisture or the stains on the linen. At first the emissions occur less frequently, afterwards two or three times a week, then every night, and even several times in the night. Gradually the semen loses its consistence, the color and smell become altered, the spermatozoa diminish in number, the semen is changed to a thin, transparent mucus, and is sometimes mixed with blood. When the disease has reached this stage, a soft or fresh bed, a full bladder or rectum, a little warm beverage, rubbing the penis against the shirt, and such like trivial causes are sufficient to cause a loss of semen.

In other cases the losses are excited by rather unusual causes, such as fancies concerning the copulation of certain animals, flies, snails, etc. Afterwards sleep is disturbed by frightful dreams, the patients are attacked with nightmare, and finally the emissions take place without any pleasurable sensation; on the contrary, they are painful. It is such emissions as these that are peculiarly debilitating.

In the day time the loss of semen generally occurs during an emission of urine or at stool—there is no erection and no thrill. At stool the semen passes off while pressure is made upon the rectum; in such cases the bowels are generally constipated, and the cause of the loss is more or less of a mechanical nature. Drops are discharged from the urethra of a grayish-white color and a peculiar odor, which, under the microscope, are found to contain spermatozoa. If the seminal fluid becomes altered, clear, colorless, thin, without any peculiar smell, the patient is generally without any suspicion. In such a case the spermatozoa have disappeared from the fluid.

If the semen passes off during an emission of urine, the loss occurs not while the urine is flowing out, but when the last drop is about to be discharged; sometimes only now and then, not with every emission of urine. In most cases the seminal loss occurs in the morning, when the urine is discharged for the first time after rising; the last drops of urine are generally thicker, viscous, ropy, adhere to the orifice of the urethra, and stain the linen like starch. If the urine is collected in a goblet, it becomes somewhat turbid, and at the bottom of the vessel we perceive small, rounded, transparent little granular bodies of various shapes.

If the seminal loss is accompanied by spinal irritation, the urine deposits in the morning and forenoon a copious, light-brown sediment; it reacts like an acid, has a sickly odor, is never entirely clear, and shows at the surface a fine, opalescent greasy pellicle, which, after removal, is invariably reproduced.

In other cases a regular seminal emission is caused by the sight of a girl, by dancing with her, by some lascivious fancy or scene, or by looking at some lascivious picture, by riding on horseback or in a carriage, by hard walking, etc. In such cases the erections and pleasurable sensations continue for a time, but disappear entirely after the disease had lasted for awhile.

One of the unavoidable consequences of this weakness is *impotence.* The quality and consistence of the semen become altered, the spermatozoa either disappear or die, or are so weak that they lose all fecundating power. Coït can only be carried on imperfectly, in consequence of the semen being expelled too soon. Gradually the erections cease altogether, owing to the increasing weakness of the penis.

The disastrous consequences of excessive seminal losses will not astonish any one who considers that the semen is the most precious and most concentrated secretion of the human organism. The production of semen takes place much more slowly than that of any other secretion in the human body. This is owing to the length of the route which the semen has to traverse, for all the seminal canals of the testicles unite into a net-work, from which the fifteen or twenty coni vasculosi Halleri pass into the larger extremity of the epididymis; if all these seminal canals were extended in one line, it would be about 1,050, and, according to the English anatomist, Monro, even 5,208 feet long. This immense length shows that it is not only difficult for the semen to be reproduced, but that its excessive use must be attended with disastrous consequences to the general organism. All the functions are affected, and the destruction of the body may even be caused by such abuses. No other functions in the body affect its normal condition as much as do the sexual functions. However, it is impossible to lay down rules in this respect which admit of no exceptions. Even the structure, constitution and mode of life of certain persons do not seem to influence the sexual powers in the least. Apparently weakly individuals will sometimes bear considerable seminal losses without any detriment to their general health, whereas, on the other hand, robust individuals are affected by a trifling expenditure of their seminal fluid.

The effects upon the spinal marrow, which is deeply involved in the sexual act, and still more in the practice of self-abuse, are likewise very different in different individuals. As soon as the irritation of the spinal marrow passes certain bounds, it becomes permanent and has a prejudicial influence upon the sexual sphere as well as upon the whole body. Volition especially, is impaired by the extreme excitability of the nervous system; the activity of the voluntary muscles is likewise affected to such an extent that all their energy may be lost and complete paralysis set in. What impairs the moral and mental condition still more than the loss of the seminal fluid, is a certain revelling in lascivious fancies, which is the more dangerous the more secretly it is indulged in, and the younger and feebler the persons who are addicted to such excesses. The higher functions of the soul are almost entirely destroyed by them, and all the purer and nobler thoughts are constantly superseded by the imagery of a libidinous imagination; this unnatural indulgence affects the sensorium, the spinal marrow, digestion and nutrition. By the time the patient is made aware of his error, all these phenomena have acquired a more intense development. The effect of these silent transgressions is the more formidable the younger the culprit, and the weaker his constitution and the desire to discontinue his evil practices. No abuse is fraught with more destructive consequences than onanism.

We will now proceed to point out the consequences of excessive seminal losses, and more particularly their debilitating influence on the various organs of the body, and above all upon the nervous system.

In the beginning of this work we made allusion to a statement emanating from Hippocrates, that such patients eat with an excellent appetite, and nevertheless grow thin.

Indeed they do have a great craving for food, and use it in large quantity, fancying that this will repair their strength; unfortunately the constant loss of semen gradually diminishes and finally destroys the power of digesting the food. The patients complain of weight in the stomach, distress, restlessness; the pulse becomes irregular, and cerebral congestions set in, the patients incline to perspire during the process of digestion, they become drowsy, unable to think or work; they experience sour and fetid eructations, the stomach is distended with gas, a rumbling, and colicky pains are experienced in the bowels, the stool becomes irregular, costiveness alternates with diarrhœa; at last the constipation becomes permanent and keeps up the seminal loss. These derangements continue to grow worse; occasionally the patients feel a little better, but they do not seem to appreciate the real cause of their trouble, or else they are too bashful to discover it to a physician. The patients lose flesh, grow sensitive to the cold, have a yellowish complexion, with blue circles around the eyes. The tone of of all the organs of the body is depressed; the voice becomes thinner, almost like that of a woman; the patient is taciturn, and the consciousness of being the author of his misery, renders his speech timid and impairs his whole activity. As the emaciation increases, the skin becomes pale-yellow, the eyes retreat into their sockets, the eyes grow dull, the muscular energies sink, the patients grow weary from the least exertion. At times a weakness of the lower limbs, bordering upon paralysis sets in. In many cases the calves lose their substance first, in consequence of which the gait becomes heavy, dragging, without energy.

Not all such patients grow thin, many of them retain their good appearance, red cheeks and all the signs of health, but they feel weak, and are tormented by many distresses which drive them to suicide.

An almost constant symptom with which such patients are affected is a constant desire for motion, notwithstanding that they feel exhausted and distressed after every exercise. The patients experience a vehement desire to change their places all the time.

In common cases the disease runs its course without any fever, unless it should be complicated with inflammatory diseases. The patients are seized with irregular chills along the spinal column, in the arms and legs; soon after they experience a sensation of warmth and throbbing in the perinæum, flushes of heat from the chest to the head and on the sides of the neck, morbid contractions of the laryngeal region with sudden stoppage of breath as if a foreign body had lodged in this region. The large vessels of the neck throb, and, on auscultating this region, we perceive the so-termed *bruit de diable*, as exists in chlorotic girls. Sometimes the patients are attacked with palpitation of the heart on taking the least exercise; the night's rest is disturbed by a tumultuous beating of the heart which either sets in spontaneously or is preceded by heavy and disturbing dreams. The palpitation of the heart is increased by both agreeable and disagreeable emotions. The patients are apt to lose their breath when walking, running, and particularly when going up stairs; a sense of emptiness, heaviness in the head and buzzing in the ears are experienced. The patients are frequently obliged to take breath and are liable to taking cold; pains and shooting stitches in various parts of the chest and back, especially in the region of the heart, often frighten the patient, and a dry cough soon develops itself. Pulmonary phthisis is very frequently the result of such disturbances.

The constant loss of animal fluids and the disturbed digestion lead to a deterioration of the blood. The blood becomes watery, loses part of its fibrine and albumen, the blood-disks diminish in number, the white globules increase to excess, and the blood is less coagulable.

Beside these derangements of the digestive organs, of the muscles, blood, lungs and heart, the nervous system is particularly affected. The cerebro-spinal axis, as well as the peripheral nerves and the organs of the senses, are involved in the disastrous effects of spermatorrhœa.

The visual power is particularly weakened. The pupil dilates, short-sightedness and diplopia set in, black or shining points hover before the eyes, even blindness may set in, the eyes are extremely sensitive to the light. If the spermatorrhœa was caused by onanism, the look becomes unsteady, erratic. The hearing loses its power of accurately distinguishing sounds; very often the patients lose their hearing entirely, and nevertheless they are troubled with a distressing sensitiveness to unpleasant sounds, were they ever so trifling. Various unpleasant noises are perceived in the ears. The taste is likewise altered; the tongue is constantly coated with a thick phlegm, rendering the mouth sticky and pappy.

In the extremities a feeling of coldness is experienced; sometimes a perfect loss of sensation takes place over a more or less extensive region. Sometimes the loss of sensation shifts from one place to another. A passing sensation of burning and heat, or a sensation as if cold air were blowing upon certain parts of the body, or as if water were dropping upon it, or as if an electric aura or stroke were passing through it, are experienced. The extremities are disposed to go to sleep, or a formication is felt in the extremities, along the back, in the lumbar region, on the thighs; the limbs suddenly start especially during sleep and shortly after falling asleep, sometimes even in the day-time while the patients are absorbed in thought.

Patients affected with spermatorrhœa, generally become languid, effeminate, pusillanimous; the power of volition is very much weakened; volition is readily excited, but it does not last, there is a lack of firmness; the patient has the best intentions, but is unable to carry them out; in the more advanced states of the disease the power of volition is entirely destroyed. The patients become diffident, sensitive, capricious, irascible; the least untoward event excites their anger, but grave insults do not seem to disturb them, they are afraid of resenting them. Towards the female sex such patients are cold, they avoid the society of females and scarcely dare look them in the face; they prefer solitude, are sad, low-spirited, melancholy; they like to indulge in glowing thoughts. They are averse to any kind of work, they loathe life and often think of killing themselves, nevertheless they are constantly tormented by a desire of recovering their health. They are constantly thinking of their condition; they observe the urine, stool, watch their digestion, and all the other functions. They show an indifference to every thing, neglect their business, and are everlastingly tormented by the thought of having lost their virile powers. Depression of spirits and hope, joy and sadness alternate in quick succession according as the involuntary losses of semen occur more or less rapidly, or according as the patients are impressed with the idea of either being better or worse. If this fitfulness of spirits should be ascribed by the patients or those around them to any other cause but the true one, itself becomes either a source of joy or grief to them, especially on comparing the present with the past. The memory is frequently impaired, and, in persons endowed with higher intellectual powers, the flight of ideas is considerably embarrassed; the imagination loses its vivacity, and the acuteness and discriminating power of the reasoning faculty are weakened.

These symptoms, although they excite legitimate suspicions of the existence of the disease, are however not sufficient to remove all doubt in reference to it. To obtain perfect certainty the physician has to convince himself that there is an actual loss of semen and that the quality of the semen is altered. The stains on the linen are positive proofs of the seminal loss in the day-time and at night. If, in consequence of the long continuance of the disease, or of the debilitated state of the patient's constitution, the semen should have become too thin and watery, the recognition of the disease by the stains on the linen would be more difficult. The difficulty of the diagnosis is greatest when the semen is discharged with the urine. This circumstance is so much the more dangerous as the weakness may continue in this way for a long time without being perceived, and as this unperceived loss implies a more deep-seated relaxation of the seminal vesicles and their excretory ducts. In such doubtful cases the urine should be examined with great care, particularly the last drops of the urine which will be found distinguished by the following characteristic phenomena: At the bottom of a transparent vesicle we perceive small little globular bodies or flocks, of a somewhat shining exterior; after filtering the liquid, these flocks and the spermatazoa remain behind on the filter. Viewed with the unarmed eye, the globules appear of different sizes and numbers; they do not dissolve even in boiling water. Alcohol, nitric acid and a solution of tannin cause them to coagulate like albumen. Inasmuch as these phenomena likewise take place when the prostatic fluid, which sometimes is discharged together with the semen, escapes alone, the use of the microscope is absolutely necessary to establish a correct diagnosis. If the alteration of the semen is considerably advanced, these flocks disappear, but the spermatazoa which are heavier than the urine, fall to the bottom of the vessel.

A valuable diagnostic is the constant formation of a number of crystals of the oxalate of lime in the urine.

An examination of the semen by means of the microscope enlightens us concerning the quality and numeral increase or decrease of the spermatozoa. If the seminal loss had lasted a long time, the spermatozoa diminish in number, are imperfectly developed, move about slowly or are quite motionless. Afterwards they shrink to one-half or one-third of their normal size. If marasmus sets in, the spermatozoa disappear entirely, and in their stead we behold shining, roundish little bodies, which are probably the heads of the extinct spermatazoa. This kind of semen is devoid of all fecundating power. If an improvement in the condition of the patient takes place, the spermatozoa reappear in the semen, and their reappearance encourages the hope of the ultimate restoration of health and of the virile powers.

As regards the treatment of this most important disease, there is no doubt that it demands the most rigid attention, both on the part of the physician and patient. For, although the ravages which this disease causes in the human system, are deep-seated and obstinate, yet, if the treatment is conducted by a physician of good sense and endowed with consciencious patience, it may terminate in most cases in recovery. I have treated a number of patients who had despaired of themselves, but who not only recovered their spirits but their health and became happy fathers of a family. Unfortunately, such patients are too often inclined to confide themselves into the hands of quacks, instead of applying to some honorable physician, who not only knows how to use physical but likewise suitable moral means of cure. Considering the high importance of this disease, I deem it proper to go into the treatment of this disease as extensively as space will permit, without omitting any complications or coincident affections.

The first duty of the physician consists in obtaining from the patient a confession of his errors, and a firm promise that he will abandon his evil practices. Until this is done no treatment can be of any avail. The patient must be given to understand, and to this end the physician should exert all his eloquence and persuasive powers, that no cure is possible unless the patient obeys the advice of his medical friends with the utmost conscienciousness. Let the patient understand that *a cure is possible*, provided the patients subject themselves to a rigorously systematic treatment.

In the first place it is of the utmost importance that the pernicious practice of self-abuse should be abandoned. Next the diet has to be regulated in the manner which will be described hereafter.

If the patient is troubled with nocturnal emissions, all spices and stimulants have to be carefully avoided, especially in the evening; all kinds of spirits, wine, brandy, tea, coffee, have likewise to be given up; in general the patient should drink very little in the evening, in order to keep the bladder tolerably empty. Before retiring to bed, the bladder and rectum should be emptied of their contents, if possible; it is likewise well to void the urine soon after rising. Inasmuch as the emissions generally take place towards morning, it is well to rise early, towards five o'clock; as a general rule it is injurious for such patients to sleep later in the morning, for the lascivious dreams generally occur towards day-break, if the patients fall asleep again after waking. The bed upon which the patient sleeps should not be too soft; horse-hair or straw mattresses, or the recently-invented hard elastic bed, are far preferable to feather-beds. The patient should not sleep on his back, but on the side. Previous to retiring the fancy should not be excited by lascivious conversation or books. All intimacy with the other sex in the evening-hours should be avoided; in general any intercourse with females, which results in sexual excitement, without gratification, is hurtful at any time. Body and mind should be occupied in an useful manner. Exercise in the open air is advantageous even in the higher forms of the disease. The nature of the diet, whether it ought to be light or nutritious, is to be determined by the attending physician, and depends in a measure upon the character of the disease. If this should be chronic inflammatory, the diet should consist of light food, such as easily digested vegetables, light farinaceous preparations, little meat, fruit, etc.; wine and beer, tea, coffee, should be avoided; water, a light lemonade, and *effervescent beverages* may be used. If the patients should be very much reduced by the disease, nutritious food may be resorted to, and even a little wine or beer may be used, but discreetly. Bathing in a river, and cold baths generally, shower-baths and wave-baths, douche, cold hip-baths, injections of cold water, are much to be commended. The cure is likewise promoted by gymnastic exercises, and by residing in the country where the scenery is beautiful and the air healthy and invigorating.

The private habits of the patient should never be lost sight of, and the ruinous consequences of self-abuse should be continually kept fresh in his soul's memory. In the case of children, judicious punishments may be resorted to, to deter them from such habits.

This dietetic and moral treatment, which we deem of great importance, we accompany with the internal use of *Carbo veget.*, *Causticum*, *China*, *Graphit.*, *Petroleum*, and *Phosphorus.*

[To these remedies may be added three agents, which I have found of great efficiency in the treatment of gastric, nervous and numerous disorders arising from the habit of self-indulgence; these agents are: *Aconite*, *Mercury*, and *Nux vomica.*

Aconite is indicated by great nervous derangements, sudden starting at the least noise, fitful mood, depression of spirits, apprehensions for the future, dizziness, intense frontal headache, either every forenoon or constantly, dryness of the mouth, coated tongue, distress in the pit of the stomach, vomiting of the ingesta, wakefulness at night, drowsiness in the day-time, nightmare, copious and exhausting emissions every night, costiveness. This agent will be found of no use in this disease, unless it is administered in the form of tincture, one or two drops of the concentrated tincture in a tumbler full of water, a teaspoonfull every three or four hours, until a decided improvement sets in.

Nux vomica may be given, one dose of the 6th att. every other night, if the patient complains of costiveness, bad taste in the mouth, soreness of the stomach, distress after eating, fulness in the pit of the stomach, constipation.

Mercurius vivus is adapted to the following symptoms: pappy mouth, thinly coated tongue, altered taste, sallow complexion, chilliness, great sensitiveness to the air, costiveness, the alvine evacuations being composed of hard balls or lumps, having a dark color. Give a powder of the third trituration every night.

Carbo veget. will be found adapted to constipation with heartburn, acidity of the stomach, distress after eating, distension of the bowels. If this agent should not relieve the patient,

Phosphorus may be substituted, especially if the nervous system seems to be very much shattered, and the patient complains of oppression on the chest, tendency to cough, pains in the chest. This medicine may be used alternately with

China, if the patient is very weak, the least exercise tires him and he is troubled with a ravenous craving for food.]

One of the most efficient remedies in this disease is electro-magnetism; indeed, I look upon it as indispensable in the treatment of this affection. I commence the treatment by first inducing, with my hand, an electro-magnetic current along the back of the patient; after a time I substitute the cylinder in the place of the hand and lastly resort to the electro-magnetic baths. The passes have to be made along the whole length of the spinal column. Sometimes I apply one pole to the perinæum, and the other one to the lumbar region. The current has to be induced very methodically. The first applications should not last longer than five minutes; afterwards every application should be increased by one or two minutes, until we gradually prolong it to about fifteen minutes, after which every succeeding application is shortened again by one minute. Already after the first days of the treatment the patient will perceive an amelioration; his apathy and his indifference to the enjoyments of life will be succeeded by a feeling of ease and physical well-being; the seminal losses will either diminish or cease entirely, and all the other morbid phenomena will gradually disappear, and the appearance of the patient will mend considerably. But even if the improvement should be ever so striking, the treatment should not be discontinued all at once, for their affection is disposed to return; it is therefore advisable to continue the treatment some two or three weeks even after the patient should seem perfectly restored; the diet should likewise be continued, although, if desired, in a modified form. It need scarcely be remarked that sexual intercourse should be enjoyed with moderation, and the vicious practice of self-abuse should never be resumed.

IV. Impotence and Sterility of the Male.

These two weaknesses, although differing in form, resemble each other in one respect: both arrest the faculty of propagating the species.

By impotence we mean an inability to exercise the act of coït. Impotence is necessarily accompanied by sterility. In sterility coït may actually take place, but there is no conception. Generally speaking impotence applies to the male, and sterility to the female.

Impotence may either be congenital or acquired; it may continue only for a period, or during a man's life-time.

The causes of impotence and sterility of the male may be general, local and relative. The general causes refer to the constitution, the composition of the blood and the state of the nervous functions. The ancient physicians were only acquainted with constitutional causes, hence their theories concerning the character of these weaknesses were incomplete and erroneous. In modern times we have discovered an increasing number of particular conditions which bear upon the development of these weaknesses, and we have succeeded in establishing a line of demarcation between the constitutional and local causes. These investigations have led to considerable improvements in the treatment of these weaknesses, to such an extent that we are now able to cure a great many cases which had to remain uncured heretofore.

Among the constitutional causes we number diseases that weaken the body with more or less rapidity, and which result in an alteration or actual toxication of the blood. Onanism is one of the most frequent causes of impotence. The action of the syphilitic virus might likewise lead to impotence in the male; in the most favorable cases this poison, if it does not produce perfect sterility, yet destroys the life of the fetus.

The inability of procuring an erection is one of the most frequent causes of impotence. This inability is frequently the consequence of onanism or of sexual excesses, especially if they had been indulged in prematurely, or it may amount to a sort of paralysis of these parts caused by irritation of the lower portion of the spine.

Generally, excessive passion during the sexual act, and the violent orgasm of the parts caused by this fierce vehemence, are the main causes of sterility in the male; on the other hand, a certain timidity in performing the act, or a certain fear that it might not be adequately performed, may lead to temporary impotence.

If the desire for an embrace is entirely wanting, all intercourse between the sexes becomes impossible. This perfect suppression of all desire sometimes exists in persons addicted to intense mental labor, or leading a secluded and exceedingly abstemious life. Long abstinence from sexual intercourse has the same effect upon the sexual passion.

Impotence is also chiefly caused by diseases of the brain and spinal marrow arising from onanism and sexual excesses, and to which we shall refer more in particular hereafter. Diseases of the urinary and sexual organs, and abdominal affections likewise weaken the sexual functions. Intoxication is an obstacle to sexual intercourse. It has been observed in Holland that drunkards are frequently affected with impotence, and among the nations of the north of Europe the abuse of spirits has likewise led to an increase of this weakness.

The sexual power is likewise affected by the age of a person. Old men generally become impotent. Some, however, preserve their virility to the age of seventy, and upwards, especially if they had been virtuous and sober men in their youth. Cato had a son at the age of eighty; Massinissa, King of the Numidians, and Abraham procreated children at the age of ninety. Self-abuse and premature excesses lead to a premature cessation of the virile powers, the semen loses its vitality, and the sexual act remains incomplete. It is supposed that the excessive use of strong black coffee and tea likewise cause debility of the sexual organs.

The local causes of impotence may be various, either purely physiological and functional, resulting in alterations of the secretions, or organic and congenital. Malformations of the sexual organs cannot be cured, and we mention them simply for the sake of completeness, and in order to caution patients against making any useless attempts at cure.

A morbid alteration of the seminal fluid is one of the chief physiological causes of sterility. The semen constitutes the most important fecundating agent on the part of the male, and its fecundizing virtues depend upon the presence of a large number of fully developed spermatozoa. If these spermatozoa are diseased, or entirely wanting, the semen loses all power of fecundating the ovum. Alterations of the semen may occur in consequence of severe, debilitating diseases, of imperfect restoration of the tissues either from deficient nutrition or imperfect digestion; or in consequence of excesses of various kinds, continued losses of animal fluids and more particularly of the seminal fluid. Sexual excesses render the renewal and perfect elimination of the seminal fluid impossible; for although the secretion of this fluid is constantly going on in the testes, the epididymis, seminal ducts and seminal vesicles do no longer contribute their share to the perfect restoration of the quality of the seminal fluid. In some persons the fluid is repaired slowly, in others more rapidly. The more frequently the semen is discharged, the more slowly is it repaired. Hence, in consequence of disease or of excessive emissions the semen loses its consistence, specific gravity, odor, color, and scarcely stiffens the linen. The microscope no longer shows a super-abundance of lively spermatozoa.

The loss of the testicles is another chief cause of sterility. As long as only one of the testicles is preserved, a sufficient quantity of semen may still be secreted to carry on the process of fecundation. Even after the removal of both testicles by an operation, a sufficient quantity of semen may remain in the vesicles for a time, to effect the fecundation of the female ovum; for castration does not destroy the faculty of procuring an erection. But after a certain period, the impotence of the castrated individual becomes perfect.

The retention of the testicles in the abdominal cavity is another cause of impotence and sterility of the male. As a general rule the testicles do not descend into the scrotum until the fetus has reached the age of seven months; if they do not descend at this period, the virile powers may be seriously impaired in after-life. In such cases both the internal and external organs are imperfectly developed, the sexual appetite is exceedingly feeble, and sterility is the natural consequence. Sometimes only one testicle descends and the other one remains in the abdominal cavity; or, instead of two, three testicles are present. Such irregularities do not prejudice the sexual faculty.

Diseases of the testicles constitute a tolerably frequent source of sterility. We have already made mention of the syphilitic sarcocele. Cancer and the medullary sarcoma of the testicles likewise extinguish the fecundating power. These disorganizations generally require to be removed by the knife, and we therefore refer to works on surgery for the details of such operations.

Tuberculosis of the testicles completely destroys the virile power. Very frequently this is an original disease; it commences in the epididymis, and thence spreads to the seminal vessels and vesicles, the prostatic gland and the lymphatic glands belonging to the sexual system. Sometimes the disease spreads still farther. It develops itself more particularly in young men affected with tuberculous dyscrasia, and addicted to sexual excesses or self-abuse.

Impotence and sterility may likewise be caused by diseases of the prostate gland, of the seminal vesicles and the ejaculatory ducts, and in general by whatever has a tendency to weaken the fecundating powers or organs, or to cause spermatorrhœa; or by paralysis of the perinæal muscles which contribute to the ejaculation of the semen.

Malformations constitute mechanical causes of impotence. If congenital, the impotence is a permanent and irremediable defect. But if merely acquired, or removable by an operation, the sexual power may often be restored by adequate treatment.

Among congenital malformations we distinguish—

1. *Smallness of the penis:* All the rest of the organs being normally developed, the penis may nevertheless remain small—in consequence of various anomalous influences—and therefore short, as is more or less the case in hypospadiasis and in male hermaphrodites whose penis is not much larger than the clitoris of the female. Evidently sexual intercourse is impossible when the male organs are shrunk to this diminutive size.

A portion of the penis has sometimes to be removed by an operation. In such cases the power of fecundating the female ovum is not always destroyed, inasmuch as a mere ejaculation of the semen against the outer pudendum is frequently sufficient to effect this result.

2. *Hypospadiasis and epispadiasis:* These defects consist in fissures of the penis or rather of the urethra. Hypospadiasis is much more frequent than epispadiasis. In the former disease the fissure occurs below, in the latter on the dorsum of the penis. The extent of the fissure is various, especially in hypospadiasis. In hypospadiasis the fissure may extend from the glans and involve only a portion of, or the whole urethra, and even the scrotum; this malformation is accompanied by a corresponding diminution of the size and shape of the penis resulting from the fissure and smallness of both the prepuce and glans. In the higher forms of this malformation the penis, by the complete absence of the prepuce, and the retreat of the penis into the fissure of the scrotum, shrinks to the size of the clitoris, and, if the fissure of the scrotum should take the outward form of a vagina, may lead one to mistake one sex for the other.

In former times such malformations were termed hermaphrodites. It was supposed that in such individuals both sexes coexisted. In his legal medicine, Metzger mentions the name of Maria Dorothea Derrier, whom some physicians, such as Hufeland and Mursinna, maintained to be a female, and others, such as Stark, Martens, Marc, a male. Malformations of this kind generally result in impotence.

3. *Atrophy of the penis* is almost always accompanied with atrophy of the testes, and always causes impotence and sterility.

4. *Apparent diminution of the size of the penis:* This takes place in large scrotal herniæ, sarcocele, hydrocele, and may occasion impotence until the disorganization is removed.

5. *Phimosis* or excessive length of the prepuce may likewise lead to impotence. If the prepuce is so long and narrow that it cannot be drawn back over the glans, the ejaculation of the semen is impeded. Circumcision may restore the fecundating faculty.

Imperfect or suppressed erections constitute a mechanical obstacle to coït. This weakness may result from abuse or in consequence of severe diseases. It may likewise be owing to a sort of paralysis of the corpora cavernosa, occasioned by too frequent and too constant compression of the same, in consequence of which their excitability is impaired and even destroyed. In such cases powerful excitants, such as cantharides, vanilla, beating with nettles, or the use of other aphrodisiaca have to be resorted to in order to procure an erection. This weakness is radically cured by the application of electro-magnetism, cold baths, douches, etc. Another obstacle to fecundation is an excessive erection of the penis, which results in a swelling of the mucous membrane of the urethra, and consequent difficulty of ejaculating the semen. A deviation of the erect penis from the true line likewise prevents its approach to the os tincæ. This defect arises from an extreme shortness and tension of the suspensory ligament of the penis, or of the frænulum; or it may arise from paralysis of one of the corpora cavernosa, or the conditions may resemble that of chordee in gonorrhœa. If the frænulum is too long, the glans is rather turned upwards, and the penis is curved with the convex side underneath; if the suspensory ligament is too short, the erect penis may almost touch the abdominal walls.

The urethra may be closed up entirely by tumors on the penis, indurations, condylomata, schirrous tumors on the glans, swellings of the prostatic gland, large calculi; such difficulties may give rise to impotence which could only be cured by the removal of the original obstacle. Strictures of the urethra may likewise impede the passage of the semen sufficiently to prevent fecundation.

Obstructions of the excretory ducts, or an abnormal alteration of their situation and direction may likewise lead to impotence. Injuries or extirpation of the spermatic duct or the seminal vesicles by cutting into the bladder through the rectum may lead to the same results. The above-mentioned obstructions cause the semen to be retained and to accumulate. Generally this takes place on one side only, the seminal duct in the spermatic cord and even the epididymis swell, and a feeling of heaviness and a dragging sensation are experienced, known to science by the name of spermatocele.

Congenital malformations of the sexual organs causing impotence and sterility, cannot be removed by art. If here weaknesses result from general debility, weakness of the sexual organs, abuse of the sexual functions, they can be cured, provided the patient sare in the hands of intelligent and experienced physicians.

Homœopathy possesses a variety of agents which have been used with the best results in these affections. The proper selection of the remedy in such cases depends, however, upon a careful investigation of the general condition of the patient and of all the symptoms characterising it. By and bye we will furnish a list of these remedies and of their symptomatic indications. Previously, however, we must make mention of an agent of which we have seen the most beautiful results in our practice, and which we have found essentially to favor the employment and action of homœopathic remedies; we allude to electro-magnetism. The negative pole is applied to the sexual organs or to the perinæum, and the positive pole to the lumbar vertebræ. In some cases we have found it advisable to pass a current through the parts while the patient was taking a bath. At the close of the work we shall go into details concerning our mode of applying electro-magnetism, and we will now furnish a list of the homœopathic agents, of which we have successfully availed ourselves in the treatment of seminal weaknesses.

Acidum muriaticum, in complete impotence, relaxation of the penis, complete absence of all erections and a sense of weakness in the parts.

Agnus castus, for frequent emissions, aversion or indifference to sexual intercourse, deficient erections.

Argentum nitricum: Deficient sexual desire, shrivelling of the genital organs.

Camphora: Weakness of the parts, want of sexual desire and erections, coldness of the parts.

Cannabis: Aversion to sexual intercourse, with coldness of the genital organs.

Colocynthis: Complete impotence, complete loss of sexual desire.

Conium maculatum: Impotence, deficient erections, imperfect or short-lasting erections.

Ignatia amara: Impotence, with a feeling of weakness in tho hips.

Lycopodium: Aversion to intercourse of several years standing, with impotence.

Magnesia carb.: Deficient erections, loss of sexual desire, aversion to intercourse, no erection even when dallying with a female.

Selenium: Impotence, with desire for coït.

Sulphur: Impotence, with amorous fancies.

Stramonium: Complete impotence.

Sabadilla: Relaxed penis, even with amorous fancies;

insensibility to sexual excitement, averson to dallying with females, diminished sexual desire.

Thuja: Indifference to female society.

V. Sterility of the Female.

Sterility occurs much more frequently in the female than in the male. The causes of sterility in the female are as various as those of impotence, and may likewise be divided into general, local, and relative causes.

Among the general causes we distinguish more particularly such as relate to the whole body, and involve the composition of the blood and the nervous energy, viz: debilitating diseases. Hence sterility of the female frequently occurs after sexual excesses, or in consequence of onanism, in which case it is accompanied by a whole series of phenomena which have been described already in the chapter on onanism. There is a certain shape and development of the female body which denote a disposition to sterility. Such women are of slender make, their extremities are coarse and angular, the sound of their voice is rough and hard, the mammæ are either wanting or imperfectly developed, the skin has a darker hue and is covered with hair in places where they generally exist in the male sex, as on the upper lip, chin, etc. Considerable fleshiness is likewise a frequent cause of sterility; a lascivious disposition and excessive intercourse likewise prevent conception, as is seen in the case of prostitutes. Females who marry either too young or too old, are likewise apt to be without children. There is scarcely a woman who is entirely devoid of sexual desire; but even if this were the case, she might yet conceive, considering that the part she performs in the sexual act, is of a more passive nature. Women in whom the sexual passion is less active, are more easily impregnated, than women with strong sexual desires. The same general diseases which cause impotence in the male, lead to sterility in the female. The same remark applies to the use of coffee, tea and other spirituous stimulants.

Among the causes of sterility which are inherent in the condition of the parts, we number functional derangements, diseases of the sexual organs, congenital malformations and anomalies preventing either the sexual act itself or the fecundation of the ovum.

Diseases of the ovaries, inflammation, dropsy, hydatids, fibrous tumors, schirrous indurations and osseous concretions of the ovaries lead to the destruction of the ova, and consequently produce sterility.

If all the ovula are destroyed, conception is, of course, no longer possible.

Not unfrequently a copious leucorrhœa is the cause of sterility. In such a case it is important to ascertain the exact locality of the leucorrhœal discharge; for, if it arises from the walls of the vagina, sterility is very seldom the result of it, unless the thick and sour mucus should interfere with the free movements of the spermatozoa. If the discharge arises from the neck or cavity of the uterus, the mucus is still thicker, glassy like albumen, stiffens the linen and has an alkaline reaction. After coming in contact with this mucus, the movements of the spermatozoa are arrested on the spot. This disease is frequently in the way of conception, but it can be removed.

There are various primary or consecutive diseases of the uterus which are still more frequent causes of sterility. In consequence of other diseases the direction of the uterus may be altered, so as to cause retro or anteversion of the uterus; the os tincæ may deviate from the normal line, so as to form an angle with the body of the uterus; prolapsus and inversion of the uterus, destructive ulcerations of the substance of the uterus, adventitious growths, such as: cysts, fibrous tumors, polypi, osseous concretions, tubercles, cancer, and frequently recurring metrorrhagiæ are more or less frequent causes of sterility.

The absence of the menstrual flow is likewise a cause of sterility, especially if this anomaly arises from diseases of the ovaries. We know that an ovum is secreted at every menstruation, and this seems to show that menstruation and formation of the ovula are intimately connected. Generally women lose their catamenia at the age of forty or forty-five years, and cease to bear children; only in a few cases women have still been impregnated after the cessation of the menses. If the menses cease prematurely in consequence of some violent emotion, a cold, etc., sterility is very frequently the consequence of such a suppression, and derangements of the general health set in, which ordinarily point to diseases of the ovaries.

It is a general rule that, if the first menses appear prematurely, they likewise cease again at an early age.

Sterility of the female is caused by a variety of malformations, either of the external or internal organs.

The external pudendum may either be entirely wanting or only imperfectly developed. Some parts of the pudendum, such as the labia or clitoris may be too small; the entrance of the vulva may be entirely obliterated or too large. The labia or clitoris may, on the other hand, be excessively lengthened, the nymphæ may be abnormally multiplied or too large and long.

The vagina may be completely or partially obliterated; it may form a cul-de-sac of various shapes and sizes, having its sacculated extremity somewhere in the interior of the vagina, or it may terminate in the urethra. It may likewise assume a hermaphroditical appearance, the clitoris being enlarged to the size of the male penis, and the other parts being comparatively smaller than in the natural state. There may be two vaginæ, or the vagina may be divided into two canals by an intermediate septum. In such a case the uterus may either be compound or single. Such a case has occurred to us some time ago. The speculum penetrated both passages, and, in each, showed an os tincæ.

Entire closure or excessive narrowness of the vagina is probably a congenital defect in most cases, but may likewise result from large ulcers and cicatrizations. This defect may either involve the whole or only a portion of the vagina.

Sometimes a second hymen is discovered in the vagina, a dense membrane which of course arrests the introduction of the semen. Tumors in or near the vagina, occasioning a contraction of the organ, likewise impede conception.

Malformations of the hymen, such as excessive hardness, thickening, abnormal growths or interstitial distentions of the hymen, may likewise oppose the fecundating process.

Defects of the uterus. Sometimes the os tincæ is closed by a membrane, by which means not only the introduction of the semen but also the discharge of the menstrual blood is prevented, so that its accumulation in the uterus and the consequent swelling of this organ may simulate pregnancy. The os tincæ may likewise be closed by plugs of mucus. A conical shape of the os tincæ is supposed to render sterility unavoidable: in such a case it is very long, pointed, and its orifice is scarcely perceptible. The uterus may likewise be entirely wanting. In such cases the vagina generally terminates like a cul-de-sac, although the general health of the patient may be excellent. Generally such a defect is accompanied by a defect or an entire absence of the ovaries.

Defects of the Fallopian tubes. In some cases their fimbriated extremities adhere to adjoining parts, in consequence of which defect they are no longer able to embrace the ovary and to receive the ovum after it had become detached. This defect is either congenital or it may arise from an inflammation of the peritoneum. The tube may be very much contracted, or it may be closed at the extremities or in the middle. Such a defect is either congenital, or it results from an inflammation of the tube, or from an excessive secretion of mucus in the tube, or from tumors existing either in or near the tube. If the tubes are entirely wanting, in such a case the ovaries are likewise wanting. The tubes may likewise be temporarily obstructed or contracted by mucus.

Beside these exceedingly important causes of sterility, which it is sometimes impossible to remove, there are other relative causes of sterility.

By relative causes we understand a variety of circumstances, which in spite of a perfect development of all the organs, nevertheless prevent conception. Such causes are, for example, antipathy or antagonism between the married partners; extreme differences of age, constitution and temperament, as when a very old man is married to a very young wife, or vice versa, a very old woman to a very young husband; or when a cold and phlegmatic husband has a wife of a very ardent temperament. Such causes are quite frequent, although it is not always easy to find them out. There are instances of sterility of five, ten or twenty years standing, and where, after this period, conception took place in consequence of a change in the outward relations of the married partners. Henry II. had no children by the Duchess of Urbain for ten years. When he was on the point of separating from his wife, his friends advised him first to consult the celebrated Doctor Fernell. "Will you make my wife a child?" asked the King, smilingly. "Sire," said the Doctor, "you will have to do that, but I will tell you how." The Doctor's advice being followed, the Queen indeed gave birth to a child, and, on this occasion, made the doctor a present of seventy thousand dollars, which was a very large sum at that period. Anna of Austria had been married to Louis XIV. for fifteen years before she had a child. Baudeloque mentions the case of a high personage who could not have any children either by his wife or his mistresses. After an absence of two years from France, his wife became pregnant, and gave birth to a boy. After this, his wife again remained without children for four years. After another absence from France, his wife again had a child. The change of climate was evidently the cause of the change in the condition of the uterus. By Baudeloque's advice he took a journey out of France once a year, and by this means he became the father of eleven children, five boys and six girls.

In former times, when sterility was noticed much more than now-a-days, aversion of one of the married partners against the other may have been a frequent cause of sterility. In those times women frequently complained before a judge that their husbands neglected to fulfil their matrimonial duties. This gave rise to the enactment, particularly in France, that the sexual act had to be executed in the presence of witnesses, in order that the ability of the husband might be proved or disproved.

This statute is said to have originated in the proposal made by a certain rake who was accused of impotence, to hold intercourse with a female in the presence of witnesses, and to prove to them that he was not afflicted with impotence. This proceeding became more or less general in the 16th century, and the ecclesiastical tribunals resorted to it by statute in all doubtful cases.

The lawyers, Guy de Chanliac and Vincent Tagereau, relate the following particulars in reference to this statute:—

According to Chanliac, husband and wife are to lie by each other in the same bed for several days and nights, in the presence of an experienced matron, appointed for that purpose by a physician employed by the authorities; this matron is to exhort both parties to caress each other, etc., and was to give them some elixir, and to fumigate their parts with some ointment made of dry vine leaves; finally she was to report to the physician what she had seen, and this one related the facts to the authorities.

Vincent Tagereau, in his discourse on impotence, states that in the suit of Treasurer de Bray, three physicians, three surgeons, and three midwives, acted as jurors. Both parties having sworn that they would honestly fulfil the matrimonial duty without interposing any obstacles, and the jurors having sworn that they would faithfully relate what had passed between the parties, these are conducted into a room where both are carefully examined, from the vertex to the feet, in order to ascertain whether there might be any natural obstacles to the sexual act; the parts of the husband were washed with tepid water, and the woman was placed for a while in a tepid bath. After this, husband and wife lie together in the same bed, the curtains are closed and the husband is requested to fulfil the act. In one or two hours the jurors are either called or they come of their own accord, and examine the female, in order to find out whether the thing had been accomplished. The proceedings are communicated to the ecclesiastical tribunal.

It often happens that women who had no children by one husband, have children by another one, and vice versa, that husbands whom their wives accused of being unable to procreate children, have children by other wives. In 1653 the Marquis de Langry married, at the age of twenty-five years, Lady Mary de Courtomier, fourteen years old, and for four years they lived together on the best understanding. In the fifth year the lady charged her husband with impotence. Experts declared that both parties were perfectly formed. The lady, however, insisted upon her charge, and the marriage, in spite of all the efforts of the Marquis to the contrary, was declared null and void. He afterwards married Diana of Montault, by whom he had seven children. Such results have occurred and will continue to occur very frequently.

We do not consider it necessary, in order that conception may take place, that the thrill should occur simultaneously in both parties, but it is a settled fact that the nearer to the menstrual period the sexual act takes place, the more certainly the women will conceive, because an ovum is already detached at this period, and is on its way to the uterus. It has likewise been observed that pregnancy takes place more readily after the parties have been separated for a while, or if they observe due moderation in the exercise of their matrimonial functions. Among the orthodox Jews the women generally bear many children, probably owing to the fact that the husband is not allowed to have any intercourse with his wife for one fortnight after her menstruation.

The treatment of this disease is pretty much the same as that of impotence. A careful examination of both parties and absolute confidence in the physician are indispensable to a cure. A variety of circumstances may sometimes operate to bring about such a condition, and unless they are known, it is impossible to remove them by treatment, provided, however, that no malformations are in the way.

The examination has to embrace the whole history of the parties themselves, and even of the parents; the sexual organs have to be subjected to a careful inspection.

It would be impossible to indicate a suitable treatment for every case of sterility; the best method is to consult an intelligent and conscientious physician, who, after taking cognizance of every circumstance bearing upon the case, will be best able to remove the difficulty.

We will mention a few general rules of treatment in order to convince interested parties that a cure is often possible.

One of the most frequent causes of sterility is weakness of the sexual organs and of the sexual functions, accompanied by general debility; the former weakness generally arises from abuse of the parts, the latter from sickness.

To remove the weakness of the organs, the patients will have to avoid for a time every thing that might excite the organs. The same diet will therefore have to be observed in sterility that has been recommended for impotence.

Homœopathic agents and electro-magnetism have likewise proved very efficient in the treatment of sterility. One pole is applied to the parts, or even introduced in the vagina: and the other to the spine, either in the lumbar region or sometimes in the region of the medulla oblongata.

The moral condition of the patient is of great importance; with reference to such symptoms, *Baryta*, *Conium*, *Dulcamara*, *Platina*, *Sepia*, or *Sulphur*, may be administered. [*Conium* more particularly when the patient inclines to sadness and is easily moved to tears by little trifles, or is disposed to feel vexed; *Platina* when the patient feels oppressed with anxiety, or feels very cheerful one day, and low-spirited the next; *Sepia*, for great sadness, disposition to find fault; *Sulphur*, for despondency, irascible disposition, forgetful.]

Congenital malformations are generally incurable. If sterility depends upon some local cause, this is frequently removeable. Diseases of the ovaries and uterus, and more particularly leucorrhœa, can be cured by proper treatment, and the sterility caused by them, will likewise yield.

For chronic ovaritis, which is such a frequent cause of sterility, we give at times *Cocculus*, at others *Ignatia*, especially if the patients complain of dull pains in the pelvic region. If the disease is of long standing, and the patients complain of dull, burning pains deep in the pelvis, *Arsenicum album* is indicated. If the inflammation had been caused by sexual excesses or by onanism, *China*, in conjunction with electro-magnetism, will prove useful. If complicated with nymphomania, *Platina*, *Sepia* or *Sulphur* may be exhibited.

Chronic affections of the uterus require: *Arsenic.*, *Cocculus*, *Nux vomica*, *Platina* and *Sepia.*

[*Arsenic.* for schirrus and carcinoma of the uterus, with burning and shooting pains, discharge of foul and corrosive sanguineous ichor;

Cocculus for uterine spasms, amenorrhœa, indurations of the cervix;

Nux vomica: chronic congestions of the uterus, with burning heat, heaviness, sticking and pressure; contractive uterine spasms, a griping and digging sensation, with discharge of clots of congealed blood; pressure towards the genital organs, early in the morning, in bed, or during a walk in the open air, with contraction in the hypogastrium; excessive duration of the menses, a constant flow, but not very copious, or paroxysmal gushes of blood;

Platina for uterine hysteria, with intolerable titillation in the uterus, or uterine disorganizations with symptoms of putrescence;

Sepia, schirrous disorganizations of the cervix, discharge of a purulent, foul matter.]

VI.—Spinal Diseases.

The spinal marrow is frequently involved in diseases of the sexual organs, especially when such diseases arise from premature or unnatural sexual excesses.

Diseases of the spinal marrow manifest themselves either as local affections, or in remote parts, most generally and first in the lower extremities, urinary bladder, sexual parts, etc. It is not our intention to furnish a complete treatise of diseases of the spine, and we shall simply confine ourselves to such as are intimately connected with the condition of the sexual organs, and either result from or give rise to a derangement of the sexual functions. It is true, scarcely any spinal disease does not exercise some influence on these functions, but there are some spinal affections that are more immediately related to the sexual sphere.

Spinal Irritation.

A pain or soreness of the spine is a frequent accompaniment of diseases of the sexual organs. It is generally in the lumbar and sacral region that the irritation of the spine is seated. It is accompanied by great excitability of the sexual organs, erections, etc. This irritation of the spinal genital nerves is generally caused by hysteria, sexual excesses, onanism, leucorrhœa, carcinoma of the womb, gonorrhœa, and urinary diseases. This kind of irritation is pretty common among the higher classes, especially that portion whose minds and bodies have been subjected to the perverse systems of education prescribed by fashion; it is known under the comprehensive appellations of hypochondria and hysteria. The symptoms are aggravated by disagreeable emotions, luxurious living, stimulating drinks, menstrual derangements, late rising, sleeping on the back, and sexual irritations.

The treatment is regulated agreeably to the primary causes of this disease. Among the general means by which the disease is removed, we distinguish: a strict diet, little or no meat, no spirituous beverages, coffee or tea, perfect avoidance of all sexual irritations; frequent exercise in which every part of the body is interested, regular and systematic gymnastic exercises, country-air, travelling, short and calm sleep, walking early in the morning, bathing in rivers, sea-bathing, hydropathic treatment, the use of electro-magnetism.

Of internal remedies we recommend: *Acid. nitr.*, *Acid. phosphor.*, *Arsenic.*, *Belladonna*, *Bryonia*, *Calcar. carb.*, *Chamom.*, *Coffea*, *Colocynth.*, *Cocculus*, *Conium*, *Causticum*, *Ferrum*, *Graphites*, *Lycop.*, *Nux vom.*, *Opium*, *Pulsat.*, *Rhus tox.*, *Sepia*, *Sulphur*, *Veratr. alb.*

[The selection of each particular agent depends in a measure upon the constitutional symptoms which characterize the spinal irritation.

Aconite is one of the most admirable remedies for spinal irritation characterized by soreness, lameness, weakness of the back, shooting, boring, twitching, wrenching or crawling pains, constant involuntary emissions, weakness of the sexual organs, deficient erections, great sensitiveness of the organs to the touch.

Acidum phosphoricum: Burning spot in the small of the back, drawing and pressing pain in the small of the back, hard swelling of the spermatic cord, loss of the sexual desire, frequent emissions.

Calcarea carbonica: weakness of the back with great nervousness, excessive sexual desire.

Chamomilla: Drawing or excessive bearing-down and pressing pain in the small of the back, down the thighs, sexual excitement with itching of the scrotum.

Cocculus: Laming and bruising pain in the small of the back, tremor in the back, itching of the scrotum, violent pain in both testicles as if bruised, increased desire for coït.

Conium: Stitches in the small of the back, with drawing through the lumbar vertebræ when standing; spasm in the back; loss of sexual desire; loss of semen after the least sexual excitement.

Lycopodium: Violent pain in the small of the back, with

stiffness, chilliness, loss of sexual desire, small, cold penis with inability to become erect.

Nux vomica: Nightly pains in the small of the back; beating pain in the small of the back, with eructations and chills; contractive pain in the small of the back; tense and sore feeling of the sacral and lumbar regions to the touch, or pain in the small of the back and knees as if bruised and contused; sudden stitch in the small of the back, when endeavoring to turn to one side, with dull pain when sitting perfectly quiet; constrictive pain in the testicles, nocturnal emissions, continued and painful erections.

Opium: The sexual desire is violently excited, with lascivious dreams and emissions.

Pulsatilla: Aching pain in the small of the back as if weary; stiffness and ulcerative pain in the small of the back; contractive pain through the small of the back, or stitching pain in the small of the back and abdomen, followed by a creeping and drawing in the head, accompanied by vanishing of sight and hearing; the back is painful and stiff as a board; the right testicle is drawn up and swollen, with swelling and tensive pain of the spermatic cord, or drawing-tensive pains from the abdomen through the spermatic cord into the testicles which hang down low; erections day and night; emissions with excited sexual desire.

Rhus tox.: Pain in the small of the back as if bruised or contused, when lying still, or sensation as if the part were pressed against a sharp edge; tympanitic swelling of the scrotum, with a good deal of itching; violent sexual desire, with emissions.

Sepia: Weakness of the small of the back, with increase of the sexual desire, and painful and violent erections.

Belladonna: Dull, distressing drawing round the whole pelvis; intense cramp-pain in the small of the back and the os coccygis, relieved by standing and walking; lancinations in the testicles, they are drawn up; nocturnal emissions without erections; perfect apathy when thinking of the other sex.]

Tabes dorsalis.

This is a disease of the spinal marrow in consequence of which the muscular energy and elasticity gradually disappear, and which, from emaciation of the long dorsal and lumbar muscles, gradually leads to general consumption and perfect paralysis.

Both sexes are liable to this disease, but more particularly young men. It is frequently overlooked in females, on account of the greater delicacy with which their condition has to be examined and inquired into. It is either the direct or indirect consequence of sexual excesses, bodily fatigue or cold. The disease is sometimes preceded for years by symptoms of increased irritability and relaxation of the sexual organs characterized by an inability to perform the sexual act, and by frequent emissions even in the day-time, and various other signs of a general irritation of the spinal marrow.

This disease commences with an unusual disposition to weariness in the lower limbs and back, and an inability to bear fatiguing exercise and to stand or stoop for a long time. After a while the muscular sensations become altered; when walking the patient fancies that he is stepping on fur or wool, and that the floor is shaking or soft; hence, when walking, he likes to stamp with the feet against the floor. Gradually the patient loses the faculty of properly using his muscles without looking; in the dark, or while his eyes are closed, he loses his sense of equlibrium, staggers to and fro, and frequently consults a physician about his vertigo. When the dorsum of the hand is extended on the table, small bodies placed in the palm of the hand, are no longer perceived by it; the patient is unable to button up his coat; all his voluntary motions are performed hastily and in an awkward manner, because they are no longer directed by the muscular sensibility and energy. The gait becomes unsteady, staggering, the knees give way from before backwards; if once under way the patient is unable to arrest his steps without holding on to something; hence he is unable to stop or to turn about suddenly, and is greatly disturbed by trifling obstacles. At last he has to be supported in walking. The ischiatic processes and the iliac bones become prominent in consequence of the emaciation of the dorsal and glutei muscles. Accompanying symptoms are: drawing and shooting pains, creeping in the lower extremities and the back; sensitiveness of the skin to currents of air; relaxation of the abdominal muscles, bladder and rectum; paralysis of the sexual organs; sweats and herpetic eruption on the perinæum; pains in the abdomen and chest, dyspnœa, palpitation of the heart, etc.

The treatment should aim above all things at removing the causes of this disease; hence all physical excitation of the sexual organs, and all lascivious fancies have to be carefully avoided in order to allow the sexual organs as much repose as possible. Spices, and stimulating food and beverages have to be avoided. The patient should sleep on a hard mattress, on the side, rise early, and never retain the urine or stool. In the first stage of the disease, gymnastic exercises, if carried on moderately and discreetly, may have favorable results. Country-air, rural occupations, etc., are likewise useful; afterwards cold baths, shower-baths, washing the chest, back and sexual organs with cold water, vapor-baths and douches on the sacral region will be found eminently useful.

The diet should be nourishing and light: milk, milk-soups, jellies, venison, etc.; whey should constitute a constant article of the patient's diet.

Internally the patient may use *Aconite*, *Acidum phosphoricum*, *Arsenicum*, *Graphites* and *Lycopodium*, especially the three first named remedies, in the order in which they are named. The cautious use of electro-magnetism is attended with the best results.

Diseases of the Urinary Organs.

These diseases frequently exist independently of syphilis or derangements of the sexual functions. They are generally painful, troublesome and dangerous diseases, the rather that many patients aggravate their condition by not applying to a physician in season. Syphilitic diseases of the urinary organs and of the prostate gland having been treated in the previous chapters, we have only to describe the symptoms and indicate the treatment of such affections of these parts as do not arise from a syphilitic cause.

I. Retention of Urine.

By retention of urine we understand an inability to void the urine. This weakness is a symptom of many urinary affections, and is frequently painful and attended with dangerous consequences; it may even endanger life, and should be attended to as soon as it is perceived.

The causes of this disease may be divided into two groups, one of which embraces all those influences which neutralize the contractile power of the bladder; and the other, such as prevent the emission of urine, although the contractile power of the bladder is perfect.

In describing the anatomy of the bladder, we showed that it is provided with muscular fibres, which enable it to contract whenever an adequate stimulus is acting upon it. This contractile power of the bladder is one of its chief means of voiding the urine, for the peritoneum and the diaphragm are only indirectly concerned in the emission of urine, and would be unable, in case the bladder were paralyzed, to expel the urine. If the bladder is no longer capable of contracting, we say that the bladder is paralyzed. This is always accompanied by a complete retention of the urine. If the contractile power of the bladder is only weakened, the retention of urine will only be imperfect.

Among the diseases which lead to the retention of urine, we number: diseases of the brain and spinal marrow; excessive distention of the muscular fibres of the bladder, which takes place whenever, from carelessness, forgetfulness, or false modesty, the urine is retained in the full bladder beyond a certain period; violent inflammation of the bladder and of the adjoining organs; catarrh of the bladder; inflammation of the peritoneum; difficult labor, during which the head of the child remains for a long time wedged in the pelvis; fibrous or schirrous disorganization of the walls of the bladder; typhus and other acute fevers, during which the patients lose their consciousness and allow the urine to accumulate in the bladder and to remain in it beyond the normal period.

During the course of the diseases which we have mentioned, the sentient nerves of the urinary bladder may become paralyzed, in consequence of which the desire to urinate would no longer be felt; or the will-power ceases to influence the muscles of the bladder, as, for instance, in affections of the brain and spinal marrow; or the muscular fibres may have become so relaxed and atrophied that they are no longer able to perform their functions with regularity. In the former case the patient ceases to be conscious of the necessity of voiding the urine, and the sphincter vesicæ, after the bladder has become full and distended, loses its controlling power, and the urine drops out during motion, like an overfilled vessel when agitated. In the latter case, the bladder has no longer the muscular energy required for the expulsion of the urine.

Complete retention of the urine in the various diseases of the kidneys, such as inflammation of the kidneys, Bright's disease, etc., occurs less frequently.

The second group of the causes of retention we class mechanical obstacles which impede the flow of urine, although the bladder may be possessed of its full contractile power. These obstacles act partially from without, compressing the urethra and the neck of the bladder, and thus preventing the urine from flowing out. In men the urine may be retained in the bladder by large hernia, swelling of the testes and scrotum, accumulation of the fæces in the rectum, or constriction of the penis by means of a cord which is tied round the part by some young men for the purpose of preventing involuntary discharges of urine in bed during sleep; it was not long since that we were called to such a case.

In the case of women, retention of urine generally sets in in the fourth month of pregnancy and during parturition; it may likewise be caused by polypi in the uterus; fibrous tumors and schirrus of the uterus; changes in the position of the uterus, such as retroversion or anteversion; curvature and prolapsus of this organ; or incrustation of a pessary in the substance of the womb.

Mechanical obstacles may likewise act from within, by closing the canal as with a plug. This may be effected by stone, gravel, coagula, hydatids, mucous plugs, or foreign bodies which had penetrated into the bladder, such as pieces of bougies, catheters, pencils, and such like objects, which children sometimes introduce into the urethra for fun, and which then glide forward into the bladder.

Other mechanical obstacles are alterations of the tissue of the urethra, such as mucous valves at the neck of the bladder; swelling of the prostate gland; strictures; absence of an orifice at the outer extremity of the urethra; closing or constriction of the prepuce; engorgements of the veins on the neck of the bladder, which very frequently co-exist with hæmorrhoidal tumors and varicocele.

We generally distinguish three degrees of retention of urine, and designate each degree by a particular name; 1, *dysuria*, the emissions of urine being simply difficult, with or without pain; 2, *strangury*, the urine being discharged only in drops, in spite of the greatest efforts; and 3, *ischuria*, or complete inability to emit urine.

The affection commences in various ways. Sometimes it sets in suddenly in all its intensity; at other times it is preceded by various kinds of distress, the stream is feebler and thinner, or the urine is discharged in drops, there is a frequent urging to urinate, and only a small quantity of urine is discharged each time.

If the retention is complete, the patient experiences a sense of heaviness in the perineal region, urging to stool without inability to gratify it, acute pains above the symphisis pubus; these pains extend as far as the kidneys and glans. These symptoms are accompanied by a feeling as if the thighs had gone to sleep; the pains are worse when walking, coughing or rising from a chair; they abate on stooping forward, because then the abdominal muscles are relaxed. There is a constant desire to pass urine, the patient is constantly agitated and in motion. All endeavors at voiding urine, are fruitless. After a while, nausea and an anxious oppression of breath set in. The face and eyes become red, palpitation of the heart, fainting, sweat and vomiting set in. The bladder fills more and more, and rises up to the pit of the stomach, forming a visible tumor which presses upon the viscera. Gradually the urine is absorbed in the circulation, a violent fever, delirium and sopor develope themselves. If the retention has reached this degree, death generally ensues either by inflammation of the bladder and other abdominal viscera developing themselves, or also in consequence of the rupture of the bladder and an effusion of urine into the abdominal cavity. The urethra may likewise get ruptured, and an infiltration of the urine into the cellular tissue may take place, causing inflammation, suppuration and even gangrene; an inevitable consequence of this suppuration are urinary fistulæ, several of which frequently make their appearance in the neigborhood of the rupture.

If the retention takes place very gradually, an enormous quantity of urine may accumulate in the bladder; it may even pass upwards into the ureters, the pelvis of the kidneys, and even enter the fine urinary ducts in these organs.

Although it is not very difficult to diagnose a retention of urine, yet an involuntary dribbling of urine may sometimes be mistaken for an inability to retain the urine, whereas, in reality, it is owing to the fact that the bladder is overfilled, and that the urine flows out, as it were, in a similar manner as any other vessel would flow over when agitated.

In order to establish a correct diagnosis, it will therefore be necessary to institute a careful examination of the case by the following means: 1, palpation of the abdomen and of the region of the bladder, in order to find out whether a firm or fluctuating tumor has developed itself any where; 2, percussion of the abdomen with the plessimeter, which, if the bladder is full, will yield a dull and faint sound in parts where a clear bowel-sound is usually heard; by means of percussion we have it in our power to determine the size of the bladder and to distinguish it from the other viscera. 3. An examination should be instituted from the rectum or the vagina, in which case the examining finger will discover a tense swelling like a bladder, and 4, a catheter may be introduced, which will at the same time alleviate and frequently remove the difficulty.

It is of the utmost importance to ascertain the real cause of the disease; for unless we know the exact cause, it would be impossible to effect a cure.

If the retention should arise from an accidental delay in not at once satisfying the desire to pass urine, a single introduction of the catheter will remove the trouble. [I have found that in such cases the application to the bowels of a bandage dipped in cold water, causes an immediate contraction of the bladder and consequent discharge of urine, without resorting to the catheter at all.—Ed].

In cases of imperfect contraction or paralysis of the bladder, the urine has to be drawn off with the catheter which is then allowed to remain for twenty-four hours in the bladder. This treatment is frequently sufficient in imperfect paralysis of the bladder such as it apt to occur in the case of old people.

The principal remedies for retention of urine arising from complete or partial paralysis of the bladder, are: *Acid. nitr.*, *Cannabis*, *Cantharides*, *Causticum*, *Clematis*, and *Pulsatilla*.

[To these remedies may be added *Aconite* and *Arsenicum*, especially if the patients are very nervous and restless, tormented by anxiety, and the urine passes off in drops, looks dark, bloody, has a strong odor. Aconite is particularly suitable to hysteric females, or in cases arising from taking cold, a sudden fright, a strain.

Cantharides may be given if the paralysis is accompanied by violent urging to urinate, and if it remains as a consequence of inflammation of the bladder or kidneys.

Pulsatilla is more particularly adapted to females or persons of mild and lymphatic temperament.]

In desperate cases electro-magnetism will be found an excellent remedy. We apply it in the following manner: A silver catheter is introduced into the bladder for the purpose of emptying it, and is allowed to remain in the bladder; a similar catheter is introduced into the rectum; both poles of the battery having been brought in contact with the extremities of the catheters, the electric currents were conveyed to the walls of the bladder. By gradually increasing the electric action, fifteen applications were frequently sufficient to cure the disease completely.

If the paralysis is caused by inflammation of the bladder, a careful homœopathic treatment will be found sufficient to cure the disease without resorting to the introduction of the catheter. This is a great advantage; for not only is the introduction of the catheter under those circumstances difficult, but it is well, if the irritation which always accompanies the introduction of the instrument, can be avoided. If fever should be present, *Aconite* will be found sufficient to subdue both the fever and the disease, and if a dull pressure or burning at the neck of the bladder should still remain behind, *Nux vomica* will remove these symptoms. Other symptoms may happen to require

Arsenicum, Baryta carbonica, Belladonna, Bryonia, Cannabis, Cantharides, Capsicum, Carbo veget., Helleborus niger, Veratrum.

Arsenicum: Great urging to urinate, the urine is burning, looks bloody.

Belladonna: Retention of stool and urine; the urine

comes off in drops, of a natural color, or else of a gold-yellow color.

Cannabis: Paralysis of the bladder; the urethra is closed with mucus and pus.

Cantharides: The urging to urinate is accompanied with great pain, icy-coldness of the hands and feet.

If the retention is owing to a spasmodic closing of the neck of the bladder, one of the following remedies has to be chosen:

Acidum phosphor., Arsenicum, Belladonna, Calcar. carbon., Carbo veg., Canthar., Conium, Graphites, Helleborus niger, Ignatia, Lycopod., Nux vomica, Platina, Pulsatilla, Staphysagria, Sulphur, Zincum.

[*Aconite:* Violent urging, anxiety, pain in the region of the bladder, congestion of blood to the head, redness of the face. If this remedy should not relieve, give

Cantharides, especially if the pains are cutting and tearing.

Arsenic.: As if the bladder were too full.

Ignatia: Sharp pressure on the bladder as from flatulence.

Nux vomica: Painful, ineffectual desire to urinate, without fever.

Pulsatilla: Ineffectual desire to urinate, in nervous, hysteric females, or persons of gentle and yielding disposition.

Sulphur: Inability to urinate, especially in children, who are troubled with worms or have been deprived of exercise.]

If the retention is owing to mechanical causes, they have to be removed: hernia have to be reduced, accumulations of fæces, tumors, and foreign bodies have to be removed; abnormal positions of the uterus have to be remedied. The mechanical manipulations which may be required for such purposes, are materially assisted by the exhibition of *Aconite, Arsenic., Belladonna, Cocculus, Ipecacuanha, Laurocerasus, Nux vomica, Sulphur* and *Veratrum.*

[*Aconite, Cocculus* and *Nux vomica* are of peculiar benefit in hernia; Aconite more particularly when inflammatory symptoms are present; in general *Aconite*, and sometimes *Coffea*, will be found indispensable adjuvants in surgical operations to quiet the nervous excitement and subdue the supervening inflammation.)

If prolapsus of the uterus is the cause of the retention, the same remedies that have been mentioned for hernia, will be found useful, and moreover: *Calcarea carb.*, *Petroleum*, *Platina* and *Pulsatilla.*

If all these remedies and manipulations should fail in removing the retention, and if the excessive distention of the bladder should threaten a rupture of this organ, in such a case the bladder will have to be punctured with a trocar, the instrument being introduced through the perinæum, or above the symphisis pubis or through the rectum, according as the surgeon may deem advisable.

Having saved the patient from immediate death, we then proceed to remove the cause of the retention; having succeeded in this, we then heal the wound as speedily as possible. If the cause cannot be removed, the artificial passage for the urine will have to be kept open; to meet such an emergency, it would be advisable to perform the operation above the pubis, because a metallic instrument could easily be retained in this region through which the urine might be discharged.

In the case of women the operation may be performed either through the vagina or above the symphisis pubis.

II. Too frequent urging to Urinate.

Although this trouble is not a disease properly speaking, yet it is a very unpleasant weakness to which old people are more particularly liable. A frequent urging to urinate, with or without actual discharge of urine, is often experienced by persons who live in a good deal of company or who lead a sedentary life. The urging increases more or less gradually, but a resistance to the desire to urinate is exceedingly distressing. If the emission of urine is postponed too long, it sometimes becomes impossible to emit a single drop, and the patient has to press upon the bladder for a long time, after which the urine comes off first in drops and finally in a continuous stream.

This abnormal desire to urinate may be perfectly painless, but it is frequently accompanied by a sense of heaviness in the region of the bladder, a peculiar sensation of muscular spasms in the perineal region, pains and burning in the neck of the bladder, contractions of the anus, and very frequently a spasmodic, periodical urging as far as the glans where a very unpleasant itching is experienced. If the patient succeeds in voiding the urine, it first passes off by fits and starts, after a while the stream become continuous, and the last drops are rather painful. In other cases there are no pains, and the patient is only troubled with frequent urging which is gratified without any pain being experienced. The affection generally developes itself gradually. After it has lasted for a while, the patients begin to feel uneasy about it and fancy that they are affected with some more deep seated trouble, such as gravel, stone, stricture of the urethra, etc., and the physician has the greatest trouble, by means of explanations and persuasive eloquence, to remove these apprehensions.

The causes of this trouble may be various. One cause may be the extreme smallness of the bladder, which, being unable to hold much urine, has to be emptied very frequently. Some persons are in the habit of voiding the urine as soon as the least desire for doing so is felt; in this way the bladder gradually loses the faculty of distension, so that it becomes unable to hold any considerable quantity of urine. One of the most frequent causes is an excessive sensitiveness of the neck of the bladder, and of the sphincter vesicæ. This portion of the bladder being naturally vascular and richly supplied with nerves, it is of course sensitive, and this sensibility admits of being considerably heightened by influences calculated to induce a determination of blood to this region. A cold, for instance, especially when arising from exposure of the feet, may give rise to an excessive urging to urinate; every body may know that a cold bath, or exposure of the feet to cold stones, increases the desire to urinate. This trouble is likewise occasioned by the excessive use of tea, black coffee, stimulating beverages and spiced food; by an inflammatory irritation of the mucous membrane of the bladder and urethra, by blennorrhœa of the urethra, irritating injections, strictures, abuse of bougies, also by the presence of stone and renal calculi; by habitual costiveness, irregularities of the intestinal canal, irritations of the rectum by piles, ascarides, etc.

Females are frequently subject to this trouble, in consequence of anomalous menstruation; acuminated condylomata in the interior or on the outside of the urethra, may likewise give rise to this affection.

The treatment should of course aim at removing the exciting cause, and regulating the diet. Tea, coffee, stimulating beverages, spiced food, have to be avoided; in general the patient should not distend the bladder by too much liquid previous to retiring to bed. The principal remedies for this weakness will be found to be

Acidum nitr., *Calcar. carb.*, *Cantharides*, *Causticum*, *Conium*, *Graphites*, *Kali carbon.*, *Lycop.*, *Natrum muriat.*, *Pulsat.*, *Sepia.*

[*Aconitum* will prove an admirable remedy for this affection, if it arises from a cold or a sudden emotion, such as fright. If Aconite should not afford any relief,

Dulcamara may be used, for similar causes.

Cantharides will help, if the urging is painful, the pain is cutting and tearing.

Pulsatilla, if the weakness is accompanied by a mucous discharge from the urethra. In chronic cases

Sepia and *Lycopodium* may be used.]

III. Incontinence of Urine, Inability to retain the Urine.

The inability to retain the urine, and the constant involuntary dribbling of the urine is a much more disagreeable, troublesome and loathsome weakness than the former. The urine passes off in drops, without any urging, sometimes without any sensation, and without interruption, or else the last-mentioned affection attains simply a higher degree of development and the bladder fills to such an extent that it flows over, as it were. In either case the sphincter vesicæ is weakened or paralyzed, and the muscular fibres of the body of the organ act so much more vigorously or alone. If the sphincter is entirely paralyzed, the urine generally passes out of the bladder as soon as it enters it.

The disease occurs most frequently among old people, or among such persons as had grown old prematurely in consequence of excessive living; the weakness of the bladder generally arises from excessive irritation of the spinal marrow, and may often be considered a symptom of incipient tabes dorsalis. In middle-aged persons the trouble may set in in consequence of diseases of the brain and spinal marrow, hernia, injuries of the vertebræ, fall of the perinæum, or during excessive intoxication, fainting, convulsions, and in hysteric persons. In some cases the weakness commences even in childhood.

This disease is not dangerous, but exceedingly disagreeable, loathsome; the clothes are soaked with urine, and a pestiferous odor of urine surrounds the patient. Such patients are a burthen to themselves and others, and have to shun all company. In spite of the greatest cleanliness they are troubled with a burning and itching, redness and soreness of the parts moistened by the urine.

A variety of this affection is nocturnal enuresis or wetting the bed, which generally occurs among children, but sometimes also among full-grown people. I have treated girls and young men of from seventeen to twenty years old for such a weakness. It arises from a relaxed state of the bladder. In some the urine escapes involuntarily in consequence of their sleeping too soundly. Such persons have to be roused two or three times in the night, in order to accustom them to regular emissions of the urine. Others fancy that they are using the chamber, whereas, in reality, they are wetting their beds; such persons should likewise be roused very frequently. There are some who from sheer laziness, prefer wetting the bed to getting up and using the chamber. In such cases punishments or exposure may have to be resorted to.

The treatment should be conformable to the particular causes of the weakness. If it depends upon other diseases, it will disappear with them. If the patients are children, they should eat and drink little at supper, and should be made to void urine previous to going to bed. Children should never sleep on their backs, but always on their sides or stomachs; for, in these positions, the urine is less apt to irritate the bladder and bring on contractions of this organ.

In the case of girls, the trouble generally continues until they get married.

If the weakness is owing to excesses, these have to be avoided, and the weakness of the sphincter vesicæ has to be removed by specific remedies.

If the weakness arises from paralysis of the sphincter, we usually apply electro-magnetism with great success, and accompany the application of this agent by the internal exhibition of *Carbo veg.*, *Causticum*, *China*, *Conium*, *Natrum muriat.*, *Petroleum*, *Rhus tox.*, *Sepia*, *Sulphur*.

[To these remedies we will add *Aconite*, *Digitalis* and *Mercurius*.

Aconite is a great remedy for this weakness, in the case of hysteric females, when the urine is quite pale and watery, or when the affection was caused by a sudden fright, a cold, or by previous, mismanaged inflammation.

Digitalis, when the weakness is accompanied by irregularity of the heart's action, dizziness, sluggish pulse.

Mercurius, watery urine, frequent urging in the day-time, costiveness, the stools being hard, lumpy, dark-colored.

China, will be found useful if the trouble was caused by excessive losses of animal fluids, onanism, sexual excesses.

Carbo veget. may be resorted to when children seem to be troubled with worms, or in case of acidity of the stomach alternating, or existing simultaneously with palpitation of the heart.

Sulphur is one of the most important remedies in this affection; in the day-time there is a constant desire to void the urine, and the patient wets his bed every night. I once treated a young man of sixteen years, who had wetted his bed every night two or three times for several years past; the urethra had expanded into a sacculated swelling, and for several months past the patient had slept on hard boards, in spite of which the urine passed off every night. He was radically and permanently cured with eight powders of the first centesimal trituration of Sulphur.] If no cure should be possible, the patient will have to wear a reservoir made of caoutchouc, into which the urine may collect.

VI. Hæmaturia, Bloody Urine.

This affection usually befalls persons of an advanced age, and men more frequently than women. The blood which is discharged together with the urine, may emanate from various portions of the uropoëtic system, the kidneys, ureters, bladder and urethra. This disease is scarcely ever an idiopathic disease, but generally a mere symptom of some other malady.

The cause may be general or local.

Among the general or constitutional causes we distinguish an alteration in the composition of the blood, as in scurvy, purpura hæmorrhagica, severe typhus, typhus putridus; or the blood may be passed with the urine in consequence of the suppression of regular discharges, such as the piles or catamenia. Some females, after their menstruation ceases, pass blood with the urine. According to Peter Frank, one half of those who are troubled with bloody urine, are addicted to intoxication. This trouble may also be one of the consequences of onanism and sexual excesses.

The local causes of hæmaturia are various: injuries of the kidneys, bladder, ureters, urethra, especially by stone or gravel; contusions and shocks in the region of the kidneys or bladder by a fall or strain; continual riding on horseback, concussion of the body in a badly contrived vehicle, over bad roads, full of ruts, violent exertions in raising a heavy load, during severe labor, coït, or when vomiting; forced marches; abuse of violent cathartics or aphrodisiaca, such as cantharides or drugs that bring on miscarriage; also vesicatories applied to the region of the kidneys or bladder, etc.

Bloody urine is passed in nephritis, or in organic diseases of the urinary passages, gravel, stone, cancer or medullary sarcoma of the kidneys or bladder, ulcerations of the bladder, varicose disorganizations of the mucous membrane of the bladder, etc.

In Bright's disease, especially in the commencement of the malady, and in scarlatina, the urine is likewise frequently bloody.

Hæmaturia is frequently preceded by congestions of the organs from which the blood proceeds, characterized by such symptoms as: heaviness, dull pain, drawing in the lumbar region and other symptoms of affections of the kidneys, if the blood proceeds from the latter organ; anomalous sensations in the region of the bladder, strangury, if the blood flows from the bladder.

If the bloody discharge is caused by injuries in the region of the kidneys or bladder, or by a fall upon the perinæum, the blood is generally pure and red provided there is no urine in the bladder at the time. From the appearance of the blood it is impossible to determine with correctness from what organ the blood proceeds. If the blood emanates from the kidneys or ureters, the blood is generally mixed with urine, and the bloody discharge is generally accompanied by the above-mentioned symptoms. If the blood comes from the bladder, the patient experiences a sense of fulness, pressure, urging and a crampy feeling in that region, a burning sensation in the urethra, erections, and if the hæmorrhage should be considerable, the extremities grow cold, the face pale, and fainting turns supervene. In such a case there is no intimate commingling of the blood and urine, and the blood is deposited on the bottom of the vessel in flocks and coagula. Very frequently these coagula fill up the bladder; and, by stopping the orifice, cause strangury and even complete retention of urine. If the difficulty arises from stone in the bladder, the first urine is generally clear, but the latter portion of the urine becomes bloody.

The urine may continue bloody even after the cause of the hæmorrhage had been removed for some days. This is owing to the fact that the dark-red fibrine of the coagula which had become lodged in the bladder, are gradually carried off by the urine. After this dark-red fibrinous matter has been removed by the urine, the remaining pale-red fibrine generally passes off in a vermicular form, giving rise to the belief that worms are discharged from the bladder.

Bloody urine is not always painful. In some cases but very little blood is passed, but sometimes the quantity is so considerable as to endanger life, especially if the hæmorrhage set in suddenly and copiously.

In treating this disease we have to consider the nature and causes of the disease. All spirituous beverages, all substances which tend to excite the sexual appetite and to bring on miscarriage, all sexual excesses, self-abuse, etc., have to be strictly avoided. If the disease is not caused by inflammation, but by sedentary habits and by obstructions in the portal system, by suppression of piles or menses, the patient should take frequent exercise in the open air in order to promote the circulation, and to remove the abdominal congestions. Stone in the bladder and calculi in the urethra have to be removed by a surgical operation.

Internally the following remedies have to be given: *Calcar. carb.*, *Cantharides*, *Mercur. sol.*, *Mezereum* and *Pulsatilla*.

[In this list the most important agent for the cure of this

affection has been omitted, and this is undoubtedly *Aconite.* I do not believe that any drug known to us is better able to remove obstructions in the portal system than Aconite, and to cure the diseases which arise from such obstructions, among which bloody urine is very commonly met with. The discharges are generally attended with a burning and stinging sensation in the urethra, and the patient is apprehensive of evil consequences, looks frightened, sallow. It is likewise adapted to the bloody urine of hysteric females, or when the discharge arises from suppression of the menses, hæmorrhoids, or from a cold. If there should be an intense, distressing and frequently-recurring urging to urinate, *Cantharides* may be tried instead of the Aconite, which, by the by, should be given in the form of tincture, and, after the distressing urging or the pains are relieved, and the urine continues slightly bloody, mixed with pus or mucus, *Pulsatilla* may be employed; these three agents will be found sufficient, to control almost every case of this disease.]

V. Gravel and Calculi in the Urinary Passages.

These are little bodies which are precipitated from the urine as it cools, and are deposited on the bottom of the vessel. Generally the deposit is composed of small crystals discernible to the naked eye. Sometimes it is a fine pulverized sediment; sometimes this sediment contains small calculi.

Generally this affection is the first degree of stone, and accompanied by gout and rheumatism.

Gravel forms in the kidneys, the finest canals in which are filled with it. Very frequently gravel only consists of urate of ammonia, with or without free urea; its color is generally red, and the urine in which it is contained, mostly reacts like an acid. There are several kinds of gravel distinguished from each other by their color, size, number, shape, surface, consistence, position and chemical constitution. Beside red gravel, we have gravel which is red-brown, yellow, brown, gray-white or ash-colored. The size varies from the finest sand to that of a pea. As regards the shape, the larger grains of gravel are at times round, at others oval, oblong, compressed in various ways, pear-shaped, cylindrical, cordiform, prismatic, etc. Their surface is at times smooth, at others facet-shaped, or rough and uneven. In regard to consistence, we observe differences depending upon the chemical constitution; at times the gravel is soft like pap, at others hard as stone. Most frequently gravel is composed of urate of ammonia, sometimes of mere urea, or of ammoniacal phosphate of magnesia, or oxalate of lime.

Some individuals are predisposed to the formation of gravel, and in others this predisposition is hereditary. Parents affected with stone or gout, generally transmit to their children a disposition to gravel or stone.

The arthritic diathesis is closely related to the formation of gravel in the kidneys; a paroxysm of gout is frequently preceded by a discharge of gravel from the urethra. Rayer observed that among one hundred gouty individuals ninety-nine were at the same time affected with gravel. In children scrofulosis and rickets seem to be allied to the formation of stone.

It has been observed that in some regions gravel and stone occur quite frequently, whereas they are almost unknown in other regions. Some have attributed the existence of these diseases in such regions to the use of sour cider and sour wine, of food containing a large quantity of nitrogen, to the nature of the water and to various other causes. But all these causes likewise exist in other places without being attended by the same consequences.

The formation of gravel, especially of the kind of which uric acid is the chief element, is undoubtedly eminently due to the mode of life of the individual. It can be shown by experiment that a rich, nitrogenized dry food increases the quantity of uric acid in the urine, whereas the contrary results from the use of simple, moderate food which contains but little nitrogen. Gravel occurs therefore most frequently among those who are addicted to rich living, to the use of meat, strong wines, etc. Patients who are affected with gravel, generally feel worse after an excess at dinner, whereas moderate living renders the disease comparatively harmless. There are substances, such as cheese, which is an indigestible article, any how—whose nitrogen greatly contributes to the formation of uric acid. Sour food and sour drinks likewise favor the development of gravel; their acid passes into the urine and thus favors the formation of uric acid.

The formation of gravel is likewise promoted by such derangements of the urinary apparatus as impede the emission of urine. Among these diseases we number principally weakness and paralysis of the bladder, swellings of the prostatic gland, strictures, a habit of retaining the urine, rest, late rising in the morning, and all such diseases as impede the freedom of motion, such as articular rheumatism, fractures of bones, etc. Women are less frequently attacked by this disease than men.

Patients who are afflicted with gravel, the chief constituent of which is an urate, frequently complain of sour, rancid eructations after dinner, sometimes of canine hunger, flatulence, costiveness, hypochondriac mood; indiscretions in eating are followed by restless nights, a feeling of malaise in the abdomen, drawing pains in the shoulders and nape of the neck. The vascular system is irritated, the pulse is full, hurried, there is headache and dizziness. Frequently pains are experienced in the lumbar region, and along the urethra; the emission of urine is accompanied by pains and spasms, and the urine contains a little blood together with the gravel. Sometimes these symptoms alternate with regular attacks of gout or piles, during which the above-mentioned symptoms abate; or else the gout and piles abate while the urine deposits the red gravel, and, after a while, again reappear. Sometimes the symptoms of gravel are confined to local affections of the urinary organs, pains in the loins which are aggravated by bodily exercise and by excesses; pains in the region of the bladder, frequent urging to urinate, itching and pain of the orifice of the urethra, discharge of blood with the urine, etc.

If the basis of the gravel is a phosphate, the constitutional symptoms are more deep-seated; the digestive functions are impaired much more, the appetite is entirely gone, the stomach is distended by flatulence, costiveness alternates with diarrhœa, the stools are fetid. Other symptoms are: general prostration, a small, feeble, and sometimes hurried pulse, extreme irritability, emaciation, cachectic appearance and depression of spirits.

The prognosis in gravel is most favorable when there is no hereditary disposition, dyscrasia, or organic disease of the kidneys or other organs; and when the formation of gravel is restrained as much as possible by suitable diet, regime and the use of remedial agents. The uriate is more easily cured than the phosphate which generally depends upon some organic disease. Gravel composed of the phosphate of lime, is the worst form of gravel, for it is generally accompanied by organic diseases of the mucous membrane of the kidneys or bladder, and by an increased secretion of mucus from these parts.

The cure of this affection is most materially assisted by strict diet, which is sometimes sufficient to arrest the formation of urates in the kidneys. We know from experience that such patients had better abstain from the use of animal food, and confine themselves to refreshing drinks, and use such bodily exercise as will promote the action of the skin. Robust persons who had lived on meat principally, will often be able to arrest the gravel-diathesis by confining themselves to vegetable diet exclusively. All heavy food, such as cheese, heavy farinacious compounds, food which is disposed to engender acids, which contains a good deal of saccharine matter, and is consequently disposed to ferment, wines, more especially sour wines, have to be avoided. The cutaneous action should be promoted by warm clothes, and frictions, by avoiding every kind of exposure to colds, by warm baths, shower-baths and by bodily exercise.

The following remedies may be used internally: *Belladonna*, *Cannabis*, *Capsicum*, *Colchicum*, *Calcar. carb.*, *Lycopod.*, *Mezereum*, *Sarsap.*, *Uva ursi.*

[*Belladonna* may be given, if the urine looks gold-yellow, the kidneys feel sore, warm, with sense of fulness and constriction.

Cannabis: Inability to pass the urine, it looks bloody, the urethra is filled with pus.

Colchicum: The disease is complicated with chronic rheumatism, gout.

Sarsaparilla: The patient had taken much mercury under alloeopathic treatment, or the urine contains a good deal of white, acrid and turbid matter, and is passed with a good deal of tenesmus.

Uva ursi: The urine contains blood and pus.]

VI. Lithiasis, Stone.

This is a more perfect degree of the former weakness; a stone arises from the gradual combination of several calculi into one coherent mass.

Calculi are generally located in the pelvis of the kidneys, in the calices and in the medullary, very rarely in the cortical substance. They are of various sizes and frequently exist several together. Sometimes these unite into one, are of various shapes, round, oval, or without any definite form, rough or smooth, etc. The chemical composition influences the form of these concretions, especially on their surface; the oxalates are generally provided with pointed elevations, the phosphates have a rough, and the urates a smooth surface.

The calculi frequently contain a nucleus of coagulated blood, of urate of ammonia or oxalate of lime, around which the remaining layers of the concretion are concentrically arranged.

The causes of lithiasis are the same as those of gravel. By inducing chronic inflammations of the urinary passages and catarrh of the bladder, calculi favor the developments of the lithiatic disease; for the mucus which is secreted in increasing quantities, causes the calculi to adhere more and more.

Foreign bodies in the bladder are very apt to become the nuclei of stones. Little fragments of pencils, needles, kernels, hair, bougies, probes, etc., are known to have become such nuclei.

Calculi, like gravel, are found in various parts of the urinary organs.

The phenomena of lithiasis are almost the same as those of gravel; only more developed and more intense, and more frequently accompanied by distressing and alarming symptoms. Colica renalis frequently occurs, if one or more calculi penetrate the orifice of the ureter and are pressed downwards into the bladder. This kind of colic may likewise be caused by violent concussions, movements, riding in a carriage or on horseback, coït, spirituous beverages, diuretics, etc., very frequently it occurs at periods when attacks of gout habitually take place in the spring and fall. The pains suddenly rise to an intense height, causing even convulsions. They do not remain confined to the lumbar region, but extend through the abdomen towards the bladder; this whole space sometimes becomes so painful that the least contact causes the patient to scream. Frequently the pains spread to the pubic and sexual regions, as far as the tip of the glans. They are generally accompanied by retention of urine and a painful urging to urinate; amid violent tenesmus only a few drops of red, black urine, which is mixed with blood and mucus, are emitted.

Beside colica renalis, lithiasis is frequently complicated with hæmaturia and nephritis.

A stone in the bladder has to be removed by means of an operation, either lithotomy or lithotrimy. For a description of these operations we refer the reader to the works on surgery.

VII. Catarrh, or Blennorrhœa of the Bladder.

This chronic affection of the bladder very frequently remains after an acute disease; it is frequently caused by other organic diseases of the bladder, prostate gland, or urethra; or it may occur as an idiopathic disease.

The most essential symptom of this disease is the secretion of a considerable quantity of mucus which is discharged from the bladder together with the urine. As long as the disease remains in its first stage of development, the urine simply appears turbid, and the mucus which is mixed up with the urine, gradually falls to the bottom of the vessel in the shape of a whitish, whitish-gray, transparent layer, whereas the urine above it clears up. Very frequently the mucus floats about in the urine in the shape of flocks and filaments. If much mucus is secreted, which is more generally the case, the urine becomes thick, the mucus is frequently white, yellow, green, and may constitute a considerable portion of the urine; it goes down as a tenacious, gelatinous, lumpy substance, which is drawn out into ropy filaments upon the urine being poured from one vessel into another. At first the urine preserves its acid reaction; as the mucus increases in quantity, the reaction becomes alkaline; from being inodorous its odor becomes ammoniacal and offensive, and decomposition takes place very rapidly. Inasmuch as the mucus goes down while the urine is in the bladder, it may happen that the urine which passes out first, is clear, and that it is only the last portions of the urine which is mixed with mucus. Sometimes the urine contains a little blood and albumen.

The emission of urine generally takes place imperfectly. Instead of flowing in a rapid and full stream, the urine passes out very slowly. Sometimes the stream is interrupted suddenly, and after many vain exertions, a plug of mucus is expelled, after which the urine flows out again more easily. At night especially the patients are roused from sleep by a desire to urinate; very often they have to urinate every half or every quarter of an hour; they feel a pain in the region of the bladder, urethra and perinæum. The urinary emission is frequently preceded by a spasm in the bladder which increases while the last drop of urine is being pressed out, and then disappears again.

If the blennorrhœa lasts for a time, the general health of the patient becomes affected; the digestion is impaired, the patients complain of constipation, pains in the loins, they have a cachectic look, grow thin, are attacked with fever in consequence of not sleeping and losing so much mucus; the lower extremities become œdematous, and general dropsy frequently sets in.

In some rare cases paralysis of the bladder takes the place of the spasm. The secretion of mucus remains unaltered, the alkaline urine flows continually, but only in drops and involuntarily from the distended bladder; very frequently symptoms of absorption of the urine into the general circulation develope themselves, and this condition may easily terminate fatally.

If the first symptoms of the disease are overlooked, a cure becomes much more difficult. Season, climate and regime have great influence upon this disease. In the summer a cure takes place much more readily, but a relapse is always a thing often to be apprehended.

The obstinacy of the disease renders the prognosis somewhat doubtful, although no actual danger exists except when paralysis of the bladder takes place or the urine is absorbed by the blood. The causes of this affection are numerous and varied. Old people are particularly liable to it. Men are more frequently affected in this way than women, especially leucophlegmatic, scrofulous and arthritic individuals; individuals addicted to an effeminate and luxurious mode of living, and to sedentary habits, to the use of spirits, or afflicted with abdominal plethora, literary men, tailors, shoemakers, etc., are particularly liable to catarrh of the bladder. The disease is quite frequent in low districts, damp regions, along the sea-coast in Holland and England.

Among the exciting causes we notice

a. Organic diseases of the bladder, prostate gland and urethra, which lead to an increased secretion of mucus in the bladder, such as: stone, ulceration and carcinoma of the bladder, swelling of the prostate gland, scrictures of the urethra, etc.

b. Irritation of the mucous membrane of the bladder by acrid urine;

c. Mechanical and chronic irritation of the bladder by frequent introductions of the catheter, attempts at lithotrimy, irritating injections into the bladder, etc.

d. Colds, and abnormal atmospheric influences, such as cold and damp air, low and marshy regions, etc.

e. Piles and gout are frequent causes of catarrh of the bladder, especially of the male sex, who are frequently troubled with this disease.

Sexual excesses, abuse of certain kinds of beverage, such as new beer, new wine, strong claret, the use of cantharides, turpentine, may likewise lead to this trouble.

A radical cure is seldom possible. An intelligent physician will therefore aim at making the patient as comfortable as possible, and prolonging his life by a carefully regulated diet and regime. Such patients should live in dry, high, sunny and airy dwellings; they have to avoid the damp morning and evening air, and in general every kind of humidity. They ought to dry their clothes well by the fire before putting them on; it is a good custom for such patients to wear flannel next to the skin in order to moderate the action of the atmospheric air upon this organ, and promote the cutaneous exhalation.

The diet may be nourishing, but it should be moderate. Spiced, salt and smoked food, sour fruit, sour, fermenting beverages have to be avoided. Fresh meat, vegetables that contain a good deal of saccharine matter, water and sugar, a little claret in water at dinner, and farinaceous food may be allowed. Pure wine and spirituous beverages should be prohibited.

The urinary secretion should be a chief point of attention with the attending physician; if it is not perfectly regular, it will have to be regulated. Before voiding the urine in the night, the patients should rise and walk up and down the room a few times in order to prevent the mucus from going to the bottom of the bladder. The habit to void the urine kneeling, should not be indulged in, inasmuch as it promotes the disease; at any rate this is the opinion of distinguished physicians. If the stream should be suddenly interrupted, the patient should not press hard, for a little shaking, or a change of position are sometimes sufficient to restore the flow. If the bladder should not be completely emptied, the remaining urine will have to be drawn off by means of a catheter, in order to prevent it from becoming alkaline and irritating the bladder still more. Catheters made of caoutchouc or gutta percha are the best for this purpose. The catheter should not be introduced too frequently, because this might likewise increase the irritation.

In the first stage of the disease, especially when frequent relapses take place, *Mercurius sol.*, *Belladonna* and *Pulsatilla* will be found excellent palliatives, and in a few rare cases *Hyoscyamus*. In the further course of the disease we have to resort to *Capsicum* and *Helleborus*. If these remedies afford but temporary relief, *Carbo veget.* may be tried. In the case of scrofulous persons *Conium*, *Dulcamara* and *Staphysagria* may be exhibited. If spasms, urging to urinate and excessive sensitivenes of the bladder supervene, *Belladonna*, *Cannabis*, *Cantharides* and *Digitalis* may prove serviceable. *Colocynthis* and *Sabina* will be found suitable to arthritic patients.

In very chronic cases *Argentum*, *Calcarea carbonica*, *Graphites*, *Lycopod.*, *Mangan. acet.*, *Magnesia muriat.*, *Natrum carbon.* may still be of some use.

VIII. Hypertrophy of the Bladder, Thickening of the Bladder, with dilatation or contraction of its cavity.

Hypertrophy of the bladder with dilatation frequently developes itself imperceptibly, so that the patient is not aware of any trouble until the urinary discharges are interfered with. The distended bladder forms a painless globular swelling above the pubes. Its exact position and the fact that it is full of urine, can be ascertained by percussion. The urging to urinate is experienced more frequently than usual, the emissions of urine become troublesome, and the stream is weaker. The bladder is never completely emptied, and, after the urine is voided, the organ remains apparently distended above the pubes, where it is felt as a tense, somewhat moveable body. The urine, especially if the bladder is at the same time affected with chronic inflammation, is turbid, purulent, and has a strong ammoniacal odor. The distended and hypertrophied bladder occasions a sense of heaviness in the pelvis, a pressure at the perinæum, on the rectum, difficulty of passing stool, a pressure on the sacral nerves, a feeling of numbness and even paralysis of the lower limbs.

In hypertrophy of the bladder with contraction, the organ scarcely holds a few ounces of urine, and the patient is unable to retain even a small quantity of this fluid; he has to pass urine every few minutes. Even after voiding the urine, the patient still feels as though the bladder were full. Even by means of the catheter but a small quantity of urine is drawn off. The urine is turbid and has a strong ammoniacal odor.

These two forms of hypertrophy, although secondary affections, yet may cause other disturbances such as catarrh of the bladder, inflammation and suppuration of the bladder, dilatation of the superior urinary passages, of the ureters, pelvis of the kidneys, gangrene of the mucous membrane of the bladder and peritonitis; some of these conditions may have a fatal termination.

The disease generally occurs among older people. The causes of hypertrophy of the muscular fibres of the bladder are frequently recurring, catarrhal irritations of the mucous membrane of the bladder, stone in the bladder, mechanical obstacles to the free emission of urine arising either from diseases of the prostate gland and urethra, or from hypertrophy or displacement of adjoining organs, carcinoma or prolapsus of the uterus, etc.; violent and repeated gonorrhœa in former years.

The treatment can only be palliative. The causes of the trouble, catarrh of the bladder, swelling of the prostate gland, strictures of the urethra, external tumors, have to be removed or palliated.

The regimen and diet should be the same as have been indicated for catarrh of the bladder.

Calcarea carb., *Carbo veget.*, *Conium*, *Euphorbium*, *Graphites*, *Lycopodium*, *Sulphur* and *Thuja* may be administered internally.

[In selecting a remedy for this disease we have to survey the whole ground covered by all the symptoms that can be traced as having had any bearing upon the existing group of morbid phenomena. If we can trace any connection between the disease of the bladder and irregularities of the heart's action, *Aconite* and *Digitalis* may prove excellent palliatives; if the affection of the bladder seems to be traceable to derangements of the mucous and glandular systems, *Mercurius vivus* and *Calcarea carb.* may be exhibited; if the vegetative system seems especially disturbed, as manifested by derangements of the digestive functions such as acidity, heartburn, costiveness, brick-dust or whitish sediment in the urine, *Calcarea* and *Carbo veget.* may prove useful. *Mercurius* and *Thuja* will be found serviceable if the hypertrophy seems connected with previous syphilitic or sycosic diseases, diseases of the prostate gland, etc.]

IX. Spasm of the Bladder.

A spasm of the bladder may either be a mere symptom characterising one of the above-mentioned diseases, or it may be an idiopathic disease, of a purely nervous character, without any organic alterations.

In the latter case it generally sets in suddenly. The patients, frequently towards the end of an urinary emission, experience a violent, constrictive pain in the region of the bladder, especially in the perinæum, which extends into the urethra, and, in the male, spreads to the superior portion of the penis towards the glans; sometimes it is accompanied by painful erections and extends to the groins, testicles and thighs. Frequently it is accompanied by painful tenesmus of the sphincter ani, involuntary stool and prolapsus of the rectum. The perinæum and lower region of the abdomen are sensitive to pressure, hot and distended. The pain which sets in in paroxysms, generally lasts only a few minutes, never more than from fifteen to thirty minutes. It is accompanied by a painful urging to urinate which cannot be satisfied. When the spasm abates, a full stream of urine is frequently emitted. On account of the excessive irritability of the bladder, it is extremely difficult to introduce the catheter. The urine is generally clear and paler than usual. A violent spasm of the bladder is accompanied by anguish, restlessness, trembling, general nervous paroxysms, cold sweat, a small and contracted pulse and vomiting.

This disease may attack persons of any age and of either sex; females, and persons of middle age are most frequently subject to it. Nervous, irritable, hypochondriac and hysteric persons are particularly predisposed for this affection.

Exciting causes are emotions, anger, mortification, exertions of the mind, irritation of the urinary and sexual organs by cantharides, diuretics, new wine and beer; retention of acrid urine in the bladder; sexual excesses, colds, sitting on damp, cold ground, etc.

The treatment of this disease has to aim at the removal of the exciting cause; at the same time we may prescribe one or more of the following remedies according to the symptoms; *Acidum phosphor.*, *Arsenicum*, *Belladonna*, *Calcar carb.*, *Cantharides*, *Carbo veget.*, *Conium*, *Graphites*, *Helleborus*, *Ignatia*, *Lycopod.*, *Nux vomica*, *Platina*, *Pulsatilla*, *Staphysagria*, *Sulphur*, *Zincum.*

[To these remedies may be added *Aconite*, when the spasm is caused by a cold, exposure to dampness, suppression of sweat, or when it is a symptom of hysteria.

Among the above-mentioned remedies, *Pulsatilla*, *Nux vomica* and *Cantharides* may be considered as chiefly adapted to this affection.

Nux vomica, when the spasm is accompanied by a painful desire to urinate.

Pulsatilla, when the spasm is characterized by a constrictive sensation in the region of the bladder, tenesmus of the bladder, with involuntary discharge of a little urine.

Cantharides, excessive urging to urinate, with cutting and tearing pain in the region of the bladder.]

It is a matter of course that the regime and diet of the patient should be regulated with great care, as in all other diseases of the urinary organs.

SYPHILISATION.

Before concluding our remarks concerning syphilis, we will allude to the method introduced in France of inoculating the syphilitic poison for the purposes of arresting the ravages of this disease; it has even been asserted that secundary syphilis has been radically cured by this means.

This method of inoculating the syphilitic virus, has been termed syphilisation, and the discussion concerning this subject is not yet closed.

For this reason we forbear expressing a critical opinion about it, and content ourselves with giving the historical outlines of this method from the commencement to the present period.

On the 30th of September, 1844, Dr. Auzias Turenne, laid before the French Academy of Sciences, a communication that he had successfully inoculated a monkey with the syphilitic virus, and on the 5th of November, 1844, such a monkey was exhibited before the Academy, and on the 20th of November another monkey to the Chirurgical Society. Dr. Auzias Turenne intended to show by his experiment that the pus of a primary syphilitic ulcer produced the same disease in animals as well as in men, and that therefore the opinion that syphilis is a disease which exclusively affects the human race, is erroneous.

By repeating these inoculations with the syphilitic virus, chancres finally ceased to be reproduced, and this gave rise to the theory that the animal was no longer susceptible to the syphilitic disease, and that the same relation obtained in the case of this animal between its constitutional condition and the syphilitic virus, as between the small-pox virus and a vaccinated individual. By transferring this theory to man, the conclusion was arrived at, that repeated inoculations of the syphilitic virus in man, produced the same insensibility to its effects, as existed in the case of the monkey, and might be resorted to as prophylactic means against the syphilitic contagion. It was afterwards supposed that such repeated inoculations might likewise be employed as curative means where the syphilitic disease had actually broken out.

On the 30th of June, 1851, the following communication from Dr. Auzias Turenne was read before the Academy of Sciences.

"On the 11th of November, last year, I informed the Academy that I had succeeded in discovering by experiments upon animals a species of prophylactic inoculation against syphilis, which I have termed syphilisation for the reason that the organism is impregnated with the syphilitic virus. I then added that experiments on man had induced me to believe that the same process would lead to the same results in his case that I had observed in the case of animals, and I have now to report that I have been unceasingly engaged since that period in verifying the results of my theory.

At this period experiments concerning this subject are being instituted in large hospitals, and some of my statements have already been confirmed. Nevertheless I deem it proper not to promulgate the facts which have been collected thus far, until they have been confirmed by abundant testimony; I will content myself with laying before the Academy the contents of a paper which was read on the 22d of May last before the academy of Turin by Dr. Casimir Sperino.

The author who was surprised at the uniformity of the results which had been obtained by both of us, undertook to repeat my experiments. For this purpose he selected fifty-two prostitutes in his wards of the hospital for syphilitic diseases, who were more or less affected either with primary or secondary syphilis. In these fifty-two cases the chancres became the less active the more frequently they were reproduced in the same individual until it finally became impossible to reproduce any. There was no exception to this rule."

Moreover it was found that serpiginous chancres, obstinate ulcers of the fauces, fluctuating buboes, figwarts and other more dangerous syphilitic phenomena, would yield to the action of the syphilitic virus if properly applied. Neither mercury nor iodine was used. This method had excited so much confidence in Turin that several prostitutes presented themselves before Dr. Sperino, in order to be syphilised, either for the purpose of being cured of the disease, or of being protected against it. "It frequently happens, says Dr. Sperino, that patients who were averse to syphilisation, now beg me to subject them to this treatment." It is attended only by a few slight inconveniences which can easily be avoided.

Sperino closes his report with the following remarks: "The question now is whether those women who are no longer susceptible to the action of the syphilitic poison, remain so for ever, or only for a time? Whether the cure of the primary and secondary syphilitic disease will prove permanent and radical? These questions can only be solved by time and careful observations.

So far it is a positive fact that all those patients who were received in our hospital for the last five months, and who were saturated by me with the syphilitic virus, have not only remained free, without an exception, from secondary symptoms, but that their general health steadily improved from the moment when the first acute chancre was produced in them, up to the time when the treatment was concluded."

"It is likewise certain that successive inoculations with the syphilitic virus remove rapidly all the primary and secondary syphilitic symptoms, and it seems to me that such results are sufficiently important to claim our most serious attention."

Sperino's observations have been conducted with remarkable tact and sagacity, and they show that no preconceived opinions should deter us from instituting similar experiments.

We will now communicate to our readers in 51 propositions the results of the method of syphilitic inoculation as explained by Dr. Auzias Turenne, in No. 48, of November, 1853; as to the value of the statements contained in these 51 propositions, we forbear expressing any opinion for the present.

1. There is but one syphilitic poison although it may emanate from various sources; but its effects vary; we may therefore adopt several degrees of syphilitic toxication.

2. An individual who is capable of resisting the action of the lower degrees of this poison, need not necessarily be capable of resisting the higher degrees.

3. All other circumstances being equal, the character of the virus descends in degree the further the process of syphilisation is carried, and the more extensive the surface from which the virus is secreted and the larger the quantity.

4. A poison which ceases to affect one person, may still be able to affect some other person who is less thoroughly syphilised, and particularly one who had not yet been inoculated at all.

5. If a perfectly healthy individual is inoculated with a poison of the higher degrees, the first chancre will be very considerable. The subsequent chancres will be less active, especially if the virus is taken from the same individual, and the pus which is secreted by these subsequent chancres, will be of an inferior quality. The more frequently the process of inoculation is repeated in the same individual, the more thoroughly the organism becomes impregnated with the syphilitic virus.

6. The virus taken from an individual that had been repeatedly inoculated, acts with less intensity not only upon the same individual, but likewise, although not to the same extent, upon others not yet inoculated.

7. This virus of a less degree is obtained by repeated inoculations of the same individual in a state of health, and, after the second or third inoculation of that same individual results in the production of the most inveterate chancre, viz: the indurated or Hunterian variety.

8. Those who believe that, at a certain period, the chancrous virus is no longer transmissible by inoculation, should have considered the double cause of this want of transmissibility.

Namely, *a*. The alteration which the chancrous virus undergoes in consequence of the process of inoculation in the same organism; *b*. The diminished sensitiveness of the organism to the homogeneous virus to be inoculated. These two circumstances lead to a perfect insensibility of the same individual to the action of its own virus.

9. Every chancre has a period of decrease during which it can be inoculated in every body in the same degree and form.

10. All inoculated chancres have the same tendency to cicatrise, and they do cicatrise provided its tendency is not neutralised by some incidental influence.

11. Chancres of the largest dimensions, which are generally likewise of longest duration, require the most time to accomplish the process of cicatrisation.

12. The extent and duration of the cicatrisation may likewise be influenced by the locality of the chancre.

13. Chancres of the same date but of different origin, in one and the same individuals, may, especially in the commencement, show entirely different degrees of vitality corresponding to the quality of the virus which had been employed for the production of the chancre.

14. Two chancres of the same origin and date, in different individuals, may exhibit different degrees of action inversely proportionate to the syphilisation which had been effected in them.

15. Later chancres produced in the same person, may be much more considerable than former ones, if the virus which caused them, is more intense.

16. Even the weakest virus is still capable of affecting persons who had never been syphilitic.

17. If a person ceases to be sensitive to the action of an inferior virus, he may still be sensitive to the action of a virus of a higher degree.

18. This virus may then still continue to produce two or three successive chancres in the same person.

19. If a person is inoculated with a virus of a higher

degree than that which is secreted from actually existing chancres, the virus which is obtained from these new chancres, is not, on this account, superior to the former virus.

20. By thus renewing the production of chancrous virus in the same person, we finally secure him completely against all syphilitic contagion.

21. The best and quickest mode of thoroughly impregnating an individual with chancrous virus, consists in effecting several successive inoculations with a very powerful and continually renewed virus; this method is, however, attended with pain, and care has to be had to prevent the chancre from becoming phagedemic.

22. The following is the best mode of syphilising a person who had never yet been syphilitic: *a.* by means of a single puncture pus of a lower degree is inoculated, after which the same person is inoculated with his own virus *every eight days, and afterwards even still more frequently*, until the person ceases to be any further affected by it; *b.* afterwards the inoculations are repeated on the same person with virus of a higher quality and at shorter intervals.

23. If a person is affected with chancre, the virus of this chancre may be taken for the purpose of inoculation, and the process may then be continued as described above.

24. For persons affected with constitutional syphilis the same process is adopted as for those who had never been tainted with syphilis, with this difference, that virus of a higher degree is substituted as soon as the lower virus ceases to act.

25. The puncture should be as direct and superficial as possible, so as to secure the smallest possible size of the chancre. The first chancrous pustule is exactly proportionate in size to the solution of continuity effected by the puncture; hence the more direct and superficial the puncture, the less extensive the chancre.

26. Syphilisation is a source of strength to the organism; it increases the appetite and the assimilative power of the organism. This method may likewise be employed against

other diseases; we know from experience that it has been advantageously resorted to against cancer.

27. Gonorrhœa and phymosis are sometimes, not always, symptomatic diseases; these are prevented by syphilisation, and they are cured in every case where the purely syphilitic character of the disease has not been replaced by an irritation of a catarrhal character.

28. They may be caused by an inferior virus as primary symptoms, in which case they may be said to be a commencement of syphilisation; or else they may be produced by a superior virus in an organism previously tainted with syphilis.

29. In the former case the inoculation may be successively repeated on the same person; in both cases persons who are not tainted, may be inoculated.

30. Venereal excesses which limit the action of the poison to a smaller number, likewise diminish its intensity. In persons who had never been tainted, chancres spread with great rapidity.

31. Chancres which do not cause constitutional syphilis, are *a.* such as are caused by an inferior virus, and are termed primary chancres; *b.* such as are produced in persons undergoing the process of syphilisation, and whose organisms have been thoroughly impregnated with the syphilitic virus; in the former case the germ is deficient, in the latter the organic susceptibility.

32. The secondary phenomena are caused by the constitutional infection, and are results of the diminished quality of the virus secreted by an indurated chancre. These secondary phenomena may be compared to the multiplied chancres of a person undergoing the process of syphilisation.

33. A person affected with constitutional chancre, cannot be inoculated with virus of an inferior quality, although a healthy person may be inoculated with it.

34. Syphilisation not being a pathological condition, it cannot be effected or transferred by injections of blood.

35. The infecting power of the chancrous virus is not proportionate to the extent of the chancre.

36. The virus of a phagedenic chancre keeps its quality as long as the chancre remains phagedenic.

37. In order to control a phagedenic chancre by syphilisation, a virus of a higher or lower quality than that of the chancre, has to be employed. A pus that can be readily absorbed, should be principally used. A pus which is not readily absórbed, assumes a phagedenic character; pus which is readily absorbed, acts as an anti-syphilitic prophylactic, the more efficiently, the higher its quality or degree.

38. The effect of this syphilitic pus is not always the same in the different stages of the chancre from which the pus is secreted.

39. After inoculation the chancre developes itself the more rapidly the more thoroughly the individual had already been subjected to the process of syphilisation.

40. The condition which, according to circumstances, is variously, and at certain periods, developed in certain individuals who had remained free from constitutional syphilis, disappears again in consequence of the successive modifications produced by subsequent chancre.

41. In order to remain perfectly free from all primary symptoms of syphilis, it is necessary to subject one's-self to a thorough process of syphilisation; this process, however, need not be carried to a very high degree if nothing else is desired than to be guarded against general syphilis.

42. Persons thoroughly inoculated with the syphilitic virus, are no longer able to produce it; the source, from which either primary or secondary symptoms spring, is drained.

43. No constitutional symptoms of syphilis result from syphilisation; on the contrary, if any such exist, they disappear in consequence.

44. A chancrous cicatrix is just as susceptible to the syphilitic virus as any other part of the skin.

45. Syphilisation is not effected locally; if one portion of the body is under the influence of the syphilitic virus, the whole body is.

46. The prophylactic effects of syphilisation are not transitory, nor are they idiosyncratic.

47. Animals are less susceptible to the syphilitic virus than men, although not all of them in the same degree. A dog, for instance, is less susceptible than a rabbit; a rabbit less than a cat; a cat less than monkeys in general; we say in general, for some monkeys are more susceptible than cats.

48. A man undergoing the process of syphilisation, passes through these various degrees of susceptibility.

49. The less an animal or man is naturally or artificially susceptible to the syphilitic virus, the more powerful the virus has to be which we use for purposes of inoculation. A non-observance of this rule is the cause of the frequent failures in attempting to inoculate men or animals, and of the secondary symptoms which have been frequently developed in men.

50. The syphilitic virus in its various degrees is the best standard by which the existing susceptibility to the syphilitic virus can be measured.

51. Syphilisation *upsets both practically and theoretically all existing theories concerning syphilis.* The opposition to the doctrine of syphilisation is directly proportionate to the amount of false theories which it does away with.

APPENDIX.

On Electro-Magnetism and its Curative Virtues in various Diseases in General and against Sexual Diseases and their Consequences in particular, according to the Method which I have followed in the Treatment of these Diseases for a number of years.

Electricity and magnetism are physical forces which, although they have been known from time immemorial, and notwithstanding the astonished progress of the physical sciences, still produce a great many inexplicable and mysterious phenomena. The wonderful properties of the electro-magnetic telegraph are known to every body, and demonstrate in the most incontrovertible manner the marvellous forces of these two imponderable substances. These forces, being known even to the physicians of the earlier ages, were employed already by them for therapeutic purposes.

The electrical machine and the Leyden battery were the first instruments of this kind that were employed for various diseases, and even for the resuscitation of persons apparently dead. But the impracticable nature of an electrical machine which could not be carried by the physician from patient to patient; the violent effects of such a machine and of the Leyden battery soon drove electricity out of the materia medica, and caused it to be abandoned entirely.

In 1790, Professor Galvani of Bologna, discovered that, while suspending frogs' legs, denuded of their integuments, from an iron railing by means of small copper hooks, these legs were thrown into brisk convulsive twitchings as often as a current of air caused them to touch the railing. He accounted for this phenomenon by supposing a peculiar fluid (a so-called animal electricity,) whom he located in the nerves and which he supposed was transmitted by the metallic bodies to the muscles at the moment when these came in contact with the iron.

Galvani's discovery led to a variety of investigations which, however, did not advance the knowledge of the cause of these phenomena, until Volta, professor at Pavia, repeated Galvani's experiments with particular care, and became convinced that the convulsions were more particularly excited when the conducting medium between the nerves and muscles consisted of two metals, the surfaces of which in those places where they were in contact with each other and with the legs of the frog, had to be metallic throughout. Volta taught that the heterogeneous metals during their contact become charged with opposite electricities, and that, after completing the circuit by means of the muscles and nerves, an electric current, as in the case of the Leyden battery, arises which convulses the legs of the frog. Electricity obtained in this manner, is called, electricity by contact, galvanism or Volta's electricity.

Galvani's discovery, and more particularly Volta's, was afterwards employed by physicians. The use of these apparatuses was at first complicated with a good many difficulties, and the knowledge of the physicians was not sufficient to draw from these new sources all the benefit they might have yielded. Physicians, being unused to such new phenomena, soon lost sight of them, and natural philosophers were the only ones who continued to investigate and apply them. The gradual elucidation of the phenomena of electricity and galvanism by means of the physical sciences is too well known to require any detailed account of it in this place. Latterly medical science again became intimately mixed up with the natural sciences, and electricity and magnetism were again resorted to for therapeutic purposes. The fact that soft iron, when surrounded by copper wire, and sufficiently insulated, is rendered magnetic by passing through it a current of electricity, led to the discovery of the electro-magnetic apparatuses in which both forces are combined and act together. Clever mechanicians simplified these apparatuses so as to render them available for purposes of cure, and to induce physicians to use them. Their expectations relative to the curative effects of these apparatuses, were surpassed in every respect.

For a number of years I have instituted experiments with

electro-magnetism, both on men and animals, and I have had abundant opportunities of verifying the extent of its curative agency. The results which I have obtained by means of the method which I am in the habit of pursuing, are so striking that I cannot forbear to give them to my readers. Previously, however, I deem it advisable to offer a few hints concerning the mode in which the electric principle acts in the animal organism, even when excited by external applications.

It is well known that at every contact of heterogeneous substances, or while different parts of the body are exposed to different degrees of temperature, or during all chemical processes, the electricity of the body with which these various processes take place, is excited into polar action; hence it is undeniable that electricity plays an important part in the living organism. During the oxydation or carbonization of the blood, during the process of digestion and so forth, electricity exercises the most important part. It is certain that many diseases, such as rheumatism, gout, etc., arise simply from the fact that the electrical condition of the part had been rendered abnormal by the local depression of the temperature of the affected part.

The Italian naturalist, Mateucci, has demonstrated the existence of electricity in the living organism by numerous experiments. According to his doctrine, however, it is not the nerves but the muscles that are the vehicles of this electric action. He asserts that the nervous principle is still enveloped in much mystery and is entirely distinct from electricity. Dubois Raymond, however, by his experiments which are described in his work on animal electricity, has refuted Mateucci in the most conclusive manner. Dubois Raymond proved by experiment that animal electricity is contained in every part of the nervous system; he shows that the nerves are capable of producing all the known phenomena of electricity, even the deviation of the magnetic needle by means of a multiplicator. He further shows that this electrical action is not simply an indifferent adjunct but an essential cause of the internal movements of the animal organism. According to this observer the electrical action is identical with the hypothetical nervous fluid.

Professor Hassenstein has likewise shown that during life a portion of the natural electricity of the animal body is constantly excited into polar action. According to him, the central organs of the nerves are the immediate causes of this action, and the nerves are its carriers and vehicles throughout the whole organism. The electric action which we see in the muscles, is a consequence of that nervous action, and, therefore, depending upon the latter.

We infer from this incontestible fact that this electrical action of the nerves must have a definite polar direction. This point has likewise been demonstrated by Hassenstein experimentally, and likewise that the polarity of this action is unchangeable, whereas formerly it was supposed that it is changeable. This electrical action differs in different individuals, but it remains nearly the same during health in the same person, and within a period of time of about the same length.

The whole surface of the body is negatively electric; this electricity is most feeble in those parts which are nearest to the central organs, and most intense in parts which are most remote from them. This fact explains the character of the polarity of the nervous electricity, and shows that the negative pole is directed towards the external, and the positive pole towards the internal surfaces. In this respect the animal body has to be looked upon as a Voltaic pile, the surface of the body constituting the negative, and the central organs the positive pole of the pile. In the same manner as the action of these electricities which now attract and then again repel each other, is kept up in the pile in a definite polar direction, is the electrical action maintained in the central nervous organs and in the nerves themselves as long as life lasts. This action ceases after death; the electricities unite and the central organs are no longer able to separate them.

From these preceding remarks we infer that only a portion

of the natural electricity of the organic body is in polar action, and that another portion remains latent. Some of this latent electricity may, however, be excited into polar action by external stimuli, and this polarity may be altered ad libitum according as the negative pole is applied to the peripheral nerves and the positive pole to the central organs, or vice versa the negative pole to the central organs and the positive pole to the peripheral nerves.

By applying the negative pole to the hand and the positive pole to the spine, the ensuing electrical induction causes a repulsion of the homogeneous and an attraction of the opposite electricities, and the polar direction of these attractions and repulsions is the opposite of what it is in the original bodies. On the contrary, if the positive pole be applied to the hand, and the negative pole to the back or the forehead, the electricity which is set free, will have the same polarity as the natural electricity. In the former case the electrical action originally existing in the nerves is diminished, in the latter case increased. It is readily perceived that in whatever body a certain amount of electricity is excited into polar action, its natural electrical action is increased when by some adequate stimulus, a larger amount of its electricity is excited into a corresponding polar action. On the contrary, if a portion of the previously latent electricity is excited into a polar action opposite to the polarity of the electricity which is already active in the part, a larger or less portion of the latter is necessarily neutralised, and the natural electricity of the body is weakened. Hence the object which we seek to attain by acting upon the human body by means of electricity, can only be:

1. *To exalt the action of the electricity which is already active in the nerves, or*

2. *To diminish this action.*

According to Hassenstein either of these ends may be attained:

a. An increase of electric action, by applying electricity of the same polarity as that which is originally active in the part.

b. A decrease of electric action, by applying electricity of an opposite polarity to that which is originally active in the nerves.

A physician is frequently called upon either to exalt or to diminish the vital action, or to reduce it to its normal condition. In every disease, no matter what its cause, the normal vital action, and of course the electric nervous action are disturbed, there is either an abnormal more or less.

In many diseases the metamorphosis of the tissues takes place much more rapidly than in a state of health. We know that, during every chemical process, and hence during the metamorphosis of the tissues, electricity is set free the more copiously the more energetically these chemical processes are carried on; for it is probable that they are determined by electrical action. If the metamorphosis be arrested, and the chemical action consequently diminished, there is of course a corresponding decrease of electric action in the nerves. This shows how intimately the condition of the body in the various diseases is connected with the electric action of the nerves, and what an important agent electricity is in the treatment of disease.

The curative action of both electricity and magnetism is increased by uniting both forces in one apparatus as is done in electro-magnetic batteries.

We have now to state in what diseases electro-magnetism is of particular benefit to patients. Numerous observations instituted by ourselves and by other physicians, have abundantly shown that,

a. An increase of electric nervous action is required in the following diseases: hypochondria and *hysteria, anæsthesia, general and local debility, weakness of the urinary and sexual organs, impotence, retention and suppression of the menses, weak stomach, constipation, weak eyes, hard hearing and deafness, paralysis of any kind.*

b. A decrease of nervous electric action, in the following affections: *rheumatic and arthritic pains, nervous headache, rheumatic and nervous toothache*, nervous pains in general, hyperaesthesia, *rheumatic swellings, podagra, white swelling of the knee, spasmodic diseases of any kind*, such as: *cardialgia, spasm of the chest, prosopalgia, epilepsy, catalepsy, chorea, cephalalgia, excessive sexual excitement, nymphomania* and *satyriasis, suppression of milk, vertigo, fever and ague, profuse menstruation.*

c. A local action of both electricities, when the nervous action is neither to be increased or decreased, and it is simply designed to excite the chemical electric action in certain localities of the organism; as in the following affections: *glandular indurations, tumors, excrescences, ulcers, schirrus, cancer, fungus hæmatodes, fungus medullaris, gangrene, primary syphilis, strictures of the urethra, fistula, dimness of the cornea, leucorrhœa, cataract.*

My mode of using electro-magnetism is based upon the doctrines of Hassenstein and Duchenne. Having for years devoted myself exclusively to the treatment of sexual diseases, I have had frequent opportunities of employing Duchenne's method of *localised galvanization*, together with Hassenstein's method. According to Duchenne's method we are enabled to electrify on the living body, the skin, muscles and nerves, alone and isolated from the adjacent tissues; in other words, to localise the curative effects of electricity, and confine them to the skin, muscles and nerves, according as the case may require.

If we simply wish to electrify the skin, and the terminal extremities of the cutaneous nerves, we apply dry conductors to the dry portions of skin that we wish to act upon. The course of the nerves has to be exactly known for this purpose. The electric action has likewise to be regulated, for it may be increased from a mere prickling and tingling to an intense pain.

These modifications are attained by means of the following manipulations:

a. *With the electric hands.*
b. *With the electric conductors.*
c. *With metallic wires.*

a. *With the electric hand.* One of the conductors is applied to the sensitive part, for example, to the spinal column, the other conductor is held by the operator in one hand, and with the dry fingers of his other hand he makes passes over the skin after it had first been dried.

This proceeding is resorted to in the case of very sensitive patients who cannot bear the direct action of even the slightest degree of electricity.

b. *Localised galvanization* by means of metallic conductors, is effected by applying one of them to a part somewhat remote from the affected region, and the other one dry to a part adjoining the affected part.

c. *Metallic wires* are applied in the same manner as the conductors, except that, in the place of one of the conductors, a metallic brush or broom is used.

The electric brush represents the highest degree of localised galvanism. If it is moved about, or the skin is struck with it, this proceeding is termed *electrical flagellation ;* if the brush is kept steadily at one spot, we term this the *electrical moxa.*

If we desire to act upon a certain muscle without affecting at the same time the superimposed tissues, Duchenne advises to moisten all the tissues situated between the conductor and the muscle in such a manner that the electrical current passes rapidly through the moistened layers and reaches the muscle without irritating the other layers. In this way the muscle is alone excited into contractions.

The same process is resorted to if we wish to act upon larger or smaller nervous trunks; but the course of the nerve has to be exactly known.

We have not followed this method exclusively, but have often combined it with Hassenstein's. In applying this method, *whenever the electric nervous action had to be increased,* as in hypochondria and hysteria, general debility caused by onanism, involuntary emissions, sexual excesses, we apply the negative pole to the back, occiput, and the positive pole to the arms, legs, or abdomen.

In *impotence* we apply the negative pole to the occiput or back, the positive pole to the perinæum.

In *local or general debility* we apply the negative pole to the back, the positive pole to the affected part.

In *suppression or retention of the menses* we apply the negative pole to the lower portion of the back, in the lumbar or sacral region, and the positive pole to the inner pudendum, even to the uterus.

In *paralysis* the negative pole is applied to the back, the positive pole to the paralysed part.

In diseases *which require a diminution of electric action*, such as spasmodic diseases, we apply the negative pole to the affected part, and the positive pole to the back.

In *excessive sexual excitement, nymphomania, satyriasis*, we apply the negative pole to the hands, perinæum, or abdomen, and the positive pole to the back or occiput.

In profuse menstruation the negative pole is applied to the abdomen, or pubes, and the positive pole to the sacral region.

The apparatuses which I use with the best effect are those of Neef, with modifications and corrections by Steinberger, according to my own indications; they are provided with a scale by means of which the increase or decrease of the electric action can be exactly regulated. The pocket apparatuses constructed by this maker, are particularly commendable both for their neatness and their correctness.

INDEX.

www.ingramcontent.com/pod-product-compliance
Lightning Source LLC
LaVergne TN
LVHW020230110826
845151LV00003B/881

* 9 7 8 1 4 2 5 5 3 1 6 2 1 *